MW00333852

Cerebral Death

A. Earl Walker, M.D.

The University of New Mexico
School of Medicine

2nd Edition

Urban & Schwarzenberg
Baltimore–Munich 1981

Urban & Schwarzenberg, Inc.
7 E. Redwood Street
Baltimore, Maryland 21202
USA

Urban & Schwarzenberg
Pettenkoferstrasse 18
D–8000 München 2
Germany

Library of Congress Cataloging in Publication Data

Walker, Arthur Earl, 1907–
    Cerebral death.

    Bibliography: p.
    1.   Brain death.   I.   Title.
RA1063.3.W34   1981   616.8'0478   80–26410
ISBN 0–8067–2142–1

ISBN 0-8067-2142-1 (Baltimore)

ISBN 3-541-72142-1 (Munich)

Preface

From ancient times, it has been apparent that when respiration and cardiac action stopped, life would cease in a few minutes. However, it was recognized that after acute respiratory arrest due to strangulation, drowning, or mechanical agents, breathing and life might be restored as long as the heart was still beating. Thus, the heart was considered the central organ of the body, and cessation of its action was synonymous with death. The development of respiratory and cardiac resuscitation measures in the middle of the twentieth century literally restored life to the heart and lungs, but might leave more sensitive organs such as the brain in a nonfunctional state. And so a person incapable of breathing and without the ability to respond may, by reason of a mechanical respirator, have a beating heart. But is that individual alive? The ramifications of this question carry serious moral, ethical, psychological, religious, and legal implications. If these apneic and comatose persons are maintained in intensive care units indefinitely, the expense mounts to such an extent that few families can afford it, especially if there is no chance of the individual returning to his or her occupation and society. Moreover, the capacity of hospitals to care for these patients becomes overtaxed. Then too, anguished relatives are sorely grieved at the sight of their loved ones being so mechanically treated.

For these reasons, physicians introduced a new concept of death based upon the demonstration of a permanently non-functional brain. This seemed a logical development. In fact, the old cardiorespiratory criteria of death (before advances in resuscitative and supportive techniques were devised to revive a heart some hours after it had ceased beating) were indirect indicators of loss of brain function, since, once breathing and cardiac action ceased, cerebral activity was invariably lost. This basis for the declaration of death has stimulated the minds of physicians, theologians, jurists and the laity. Through constitutional law and judicial edict, the concept has been gradually accepted as the basis for the pronouncement of death under certain circumstances. As the general public has had more first hand acquaintance with the special advantages of declaring death in hopeless and comatose cases on the basis of a nonfunctional brain, it has gained an uneasy recognition in the community. Many people still view with suspicion any declaration of death not based upon the traditional cessation of cardiac activity; to them, a beating heart is incompatible with death. In most cases, this stems from the difficulty in differentiating the process of dying from the fact of death.

The transition from a cardiac based death to a cerebral oriented death has been retarded by the failure of professionals to understand certain fundamental principles and to agree upon the criteria that are necessary to establish the death of the brain. In addition, the need of viable organs for transplant has introduced ethical and legal questions related to the discontinuance of resuscitative measures. The publicity given these unresolved issues in the lay press and professional publications have confused the public and, at times, led to a mistrust of the medical profession.

For some years the author has had an interest in the subject of brain death. In the care of neurosurgical patients, the determination of brain death was often an important consideration to avert prolonged grief of relatives and expensive cardiopulmonary support when meaningful life had already ceased. The decision that cerebral death had occurred became even more pertinent when transplant surgery developed and donor organs were required as early as possible. When in 1971 the National Institute of Neurological Diseases and Stroke (NINDS) initiated a collaborative effort involving nine cooperating centers to study the problems of cerebral death, the author, as coordinator, had an opportunity to review and analyze the data from that program (493).

The views of the author have evolved not only from reading medical literature but from deliberations of committee meetings, formal presentations of scientific symposia and conferences, and informal discussions with physicians, lawyers, clergy, and other intellectuals interested and knowledgeable in the phenomena of death. It is of course impossible to identify or to acknowledge all those individuals who have enlightened the author and so contributed to the opinions expressed in this monograph. However, the author must express his appreciation of the stimulating conferences with all those associated with the Cerebral Death program which was sponsored by the National Institute of Neurological and Communicative Disorders and Stroke. In particular, the project directors and consultants to the program freely contributed their wide experience in their specialized interests. In electroencephalography, I acknowledge the cooperation of the authors of the *Atlas of Electroencephalogaphy in Coma and Cerebral Death*. Regarding computerized EEG techniques, I have consulted and derived much from the discussions and writings of Dr. R. G. Bickford and his associates. Much of the statistical analysis was made with computerized techniques by Dr. Earl Diamond, to whom I am grateful. My discussions with Dr. Gaetano F. Molinari clarified some clinical concepts of cerebral death. However, the opinions expressed in this monograph are those of the author, and should not be considered necessarily to reflect the views of the NINCDS or of other members of the Cerebral Death program.

It is a pleasure to acknowledge my indebtedness to my secretaries—Ms. Donna Dionne, Irma Ingram and Cynthia Anderson—who have patiently and graciously tolerated my many alterations that forced them to monotonously retype page after page of manuscript.

Certain specific acknowledgements are gratefully made for permission to use previously published or unpublished material:

To Williams and Wilkins for permission to republish figures from my earlier papers in *Current Medical Digest* and *Journal of Neuropathology and Experimental Neurology* (Figures V–1, V–6, V–7, VI–3, VI–4, and VI–5).

To Dr. S. Uematsu for permission to publish Fig. III–1.

To Dr. Schlesinger for permission to publish Fig. III–1.

To Dr. E. Neidermeyer for electroencephalograms of Chapter V.

To Dr. Paul Turner for permission to publish Fig. VII–1.

In the first edition of this book, the superb cooperation of the publishers, Professional Information Library, in particular Mr. Tom Pfeil and Mr. William E. Barton, eliminated much of the tedious editorial work and made the compilation of the final production a pleasure.

In this second edition of Cerebral Death, not only the new developments in diagnosis of a dead brain, but the response of the laity and the professions to the changing concepts of death receive special attention. Although the basic concepts of cerebral death have gained general acceptance, there are many ramifications of the problem of cerebral death that are just now being brought to the attention of the public. Their resolution will require drastic changes in the conceptualization of life and death.

June, 1980

A. EARL WALKER

Contents

Chapter I

Introduction to the General Problem

Introduction

Although death is not a popular topic of conversation, it has been receiving more and more attention as people have become preoccupied with health. The cessation of life—dying—thought throughout the ages to be a simple transition, is now recognized as a complex process involving a number of stages, from some of which a return to life is possible. The tissues of the body, when deprived of nutritive fluids by circulatory failure, undergo chemical degradation at different rates. Thus, under normal environmental circumstances, cessation of the cerebral blood flow for just a few minutes so severely depletes the available oxygen in the brain that anaerobic metabolism ensues and causes irreversible changes. On the other hand, the heart, liver and kidneys may recover after some period of oxygen deprivation due to a lack of circulation. Of course, if the period becomes unduly prolonged, these organs, too, undergo changes that not even the best resuscitative measures can reverse.

Knowledge of this sequence of events became of practical significance just after the middle of the twentieth century, when physicians turned their attention and ingenuity to developing resuscitative techniques that would provide basic life support for individuals in comatose states. Improved artificial respirators and external cardiac massage, which stimulated an asystolic heart to beat again, provided the means to maintain pulmonary and cardiac activity that in turn sustained the other vital functions of the body. Unfortunately, however, the application of these resuscitative measures was at times so delayed that the brain was destroyed in part or in whole by the anoxia. The resultant states of coma were the subjects of a number of papers and symposia in which French neurologists (331) played major roles. To describe the state between life and death, the term *coma dépassé* was coined on the wards of Professor Mollaret at the Claude Bernard Hospital in Paris (332). It designated a condition beyond deep coma, in which even the vegetative functions were lost and which was thought to be associated with a dead brain (510).

This anomalous situation—a dead brain in a living body—was capitalized upon by transplant surgeons who saw in these beating-heart cadavers the well-preserved organs they needed. But a new dimension in the concept of death was needed so that these persons could be declared dead and their organs removed. In the 1960s, the notion that life might be declared at an end when the brain, the essence of human existence, was permanently and completely damaged was just gaining acceptance. The necessity of crystalizing this viewpoint and of defining its medical criteria became increasingly evident as the growing number of persons being maintained by artificial ventilation and alimentation filled hospital beds as comatose patients, and preoccupied the time and special skills of highly trained nursing personnel.

Definition

Death. It is quite understandable that many primitive peoples did not regard death as a natural phenomenon, for rarely did they live to a ripe old age. If a savage or primitive man died without being wounded, he was often considered to be the victim of sorcerers and the evil spirits with which they were associated. In some parts of Africa, even today, one's death is ascribed to the magicians of some hostile tribe or to the malicious act of a neighbor.

The notion that biological death relates to a life cycle has developed in the last few centuries. The general impression is that life consists of a stage of growth, a prime period, senescence and death. However, it may be true, as some primitive people aver, that death is not a necessary and inevitable consequence of life. Protozoa, under experimental conditions, may reproduce by simple fissions of the body, so that one individual becomes two, each of which is a complete organism. In multicellular organisms, however, only the germ cells pass on genetic material to an ovum, which develops into a new organism. Nevertheless, certain fish will continue to grow indefinitely and might be immortal except for accidental or environmental death. Hence, senescence and death may be artifacts of the external or internal enviromnent.

In Webster's *New International Dictionary* (505), death is defined as "the cessation of all vital functions without the capability of resuscitation in animals or plants." *Gould's Medical Dictionary* (157) has a similar definition: "cessation of all vital functions in a living organism." The significant and undefined words in these definitions are "vital functions." It is noteworthy that death is related to the cessation of function and not primarily to the destruction of tissues, organs or bodies. Thus, the essence of life is physiological integrity, and so the essence of death is, firstly, the abolition of function. Molecular destruction may occur either before or after death—in fact, at times, long after cessation of biological function. Consider that Hogue (188) has grown neuronal and glial cells in tissue culture from brain several weeks after its removal from the calvarium. Secondly, the function must be vital, i.e., related or essential to life. In man, until recently, vital functions were assumed to be respiratory and cardiac activity, but this heart-lung notion is being replaced by a brain-oriented concept. However, the corporeal basis of this hypothesis has been challenged by some philosophers, physiologists and physicians who argue that death is a philosophical and not a somatomedical issue. In this vein, Bergen (43), in discussing the legal regulation of heart transplants, states that "philosophically, death might be defined as the point at which the deterioration of functions becomes irreversible so that the organism can never again function as an integrated, rational organ." Negovsky, a Russian physiologist, comes to a very similar conclusion, namely, that "death of a living organism is the disintegration of its unity, interruption of interrelationships of organs and systems, both with each other and with the external environment" (344). Human death is to be considered not the destruction of tissue, although that may occur, but rather an abstraction that symbolizes the transition from a biological to a physical state. Thus, in death the individual loses those essences that characterize a human being. As a basis for this viewpoint, Veath (477) defines death as "the irreversible loss of that which is essentially significant to the nature of man." These faculties include the capability of experiencing, of integrating experiences (into memory, emotional reactions, reasoning, judgment and personality), of rationalizing, of modulating and interrelating body functions and of indulging in social interrelationships. It is obvious that a lexical definition of death cannot be formulated which will satisfy the diverse connotations required by peoples of varying professions and backgrounds. At times, death is qualified as biological death, brain death, cardiac death, cerebral death, clinical death, cognitive death, cortical death, cytological (cellular) death, dissociated cerebral death, functional death, heart death, irreversible death, legal death, medical death, physiological death, psychosocial death, scientific death, spiritual death, suspended death, tissue death or virtual death.

Thus, Morison (336) has emphasized that the abstraction "death" cannot be accurately defined. To avoid this dilemma, Kass (234) differentiates the concept "death" from "the operations used to define and measure it."

However, the question still remains as to what may be considered the "vital functions" of the brain if the latter is to be the focus for the determination of death. Are these functions the maintenance and support of the organs that keep a person vegetating, or are they the more sophisticated roles of providing individuals with qualities that are recognized as characteristic of human existence? From the sociological standpoint, one may argue that a vegetative existence is not human life and that individuals so surviving are dead in that they are not capable of interacting as human beings. In discussing death with the general population, one must consider the attitudes and beliefs of the public, who, in spite of increasing interest in health matters, do not fully understand even the basic principles of medicine. The public has been brought up to believe that heart action and respiration are signs of life and that their absence indicates death. Now, within the past decade or so, the medical profession has been proclaiming that a person can have a heart that beats and lungs that respire and still be dead. No wonder that the layman's credulity has been strained to accept this proposition.

Obviously, a working definition of cerebral death is necessary. A simple statement that cerebral death is the permanent loss of function of the brain is open to the criticism that the means of determining function are not specified and so the accuracy of the definition is unkown. Is this to be a simple bedside clinical examination or a depth electrographic study? Perhaps the definition suggested by the American Bar Association—"a human body with irreversible cessation of brain function, according to the usual and customary standards of medical practice, shall be considered dead" (10)—would ensure minimal standards for examination of brain function, yet leave to the discretion of the physician the decision as to how detailed and complicated an examination would be necessary to assure that the brain was nonfunctional. In this definition, "brain function" refers to the intergrated (not isolated cellular) activity of the nervous tissue contained within the intracranial cavity.

Terminology Related to Brain-oriented Death

The original descriptions of Mollaret (330) referred to a clinical state, "coma dépassé." The French term, although an abstraction, had several advantages, namely, that the condition was a clinical, not a pathological entity, that the term had no other associated or conflicting connotations and that it did not relate to specific anatomical lesions. "Irreversible coma" as the anglicized equivalent was an unfortunate choice for it lacked the connotation of the French phrase relating to total loss of neural function. Rather, it described a number of comatose states in addition to coma dépassé that were characterized by cerebral unresponsivity but in which such brainstem functions as respiration might still be present.

However, more pathologically minded neurologists preferred a name with morphological connotations, and so the terms cerebral death and brain death were introduced. As the variegated picture of this state unfolded, some investigators attempted to make more precise anatomico-pathological diagnoses. Although a number of authors have referred to partial death or levels of brain death, such terms seem inappropriate. In most such cases, the patient is neurologically handicapped, but the state would not meet the definition of "cessation of all vital functions" even if "vital" were limited to qualities that characterize a human being, a concept foreign to the thinking of most people. Neocortical death has been described as destruction of the cerebral mantle. Destruction of both cerebral hemispheres exclusive of the brainstem and cerebellum has been termed cerebral death. Even brainstem death was considered a specific entity (252). However, although the mechanisms for experiential and social interaction might be destroyed by such lesions, respiration and vasomotor functions would persist. Should such a vegetating body be considered dead medically and legally?

Certain German writers (232) argue that cortical death alone is not sufficient to deprive a person of his or her rights as a living individual. They contend that some low psychic activity may be present in brainstem preparations. On the other hand, Korein writes "if the cerebrum per se is irreversibly destroyed bilaterally, continuing viability of the remaining infratentorial portions of the brain makes no contribution to continuing significant function of the total human organism" (250). Then the issue is whether such a vegetating body without responsivity or apparent mentation is alive. Based upon the current concepts of life, most physicians and jurists consider that, legally, life exists. Certainly, to give the appellation "death" to such states is inappropriate. Moreover, although clinically the neurological disturbances may seem to be confined to the cerebral hemispheres, postmortem examination of neocortical death cases has shown severe changes in the basal ganglia, thalami, cerebellum and, to a lesser extent, the brainstem. Consequently, it would seem wise to classify these cases clinically as syndromes—alpha coma, locked-in syndrome, etc.—rather than to designate them as anatomically localized death. It may be, as the social consciousness changes, that the vital functions of the brain may come to be identified as psychosocial, in which event vegetative activity of the body would not be construed to constitute human life. But the problems related to psychosocial death are so delicate and so imponderable that the issue does not merit further consideration at a time when public opinion barely accepts the concept of cerebral death.

Whether the dead brain syndrome should be designated as cerebral or brain death has occasioned some difference of opinion. When some patients were reported with persistent coma and isoelectric EEGs, but with retained brainstem reflexes (especially respiration), it was suggested that the term "cerebral death" should be applied to these cases and the term "brain death" reserved for total destruction of the neural elements within the cranium. To apply the term "death" to a state in which an individual, although comatose, breathes and may be sustained indefinitely, seems quite inappropriate. Moreover, the Oxford Universal Dictionary defines cerebral as "pertaining or relating to the brain", and brain as "formerly related to the anterior portion (cerebrum) as opposed to the posterior (cerebellar) and now used for the entire organ". Consequently, in this monograph, the terms "cerebral death" and "brain death" will be used synonymously to designate permanent loss of all functions mediated by intracranial neural structures. Since names similar to cerebral or brain death have been generally accepted in other languages—Hirntod, la mort du cerveau, mort cérébrale, Hjärndöd—it would seem desirable to retain the holistic designation.

Misconceptions

Given this definition, some previous misconceptions and inappropriate usage of terms require clarification.

The use of "brain death" or "cerebral death" to mean the death not only of the brain but also of the individual differs from the connotation of liver death and kidney death, which refer to dysfunctions of these organs that result in cardiac death. In other words, cerebral death *is* the demise of the individual, whereas organ death *leads* to the extinction of life.

A second problem stems from the loose use of certain terms, particularly cerebral or brain death and irreversible coma. "Cerebral death" implies total and permanent abolition of brain function so that both volitional and reflex evidences of responsivity are absent. "Irreversible coma" refers to a state in which all functions attributed to the cerebrum that identify the human essence—mind, personality, behavior and, in theological terms, the soul—are lost but certain functions that regulate respiration, temperature, blood pressure or other neuronal activity may remain to some degree. In such cases, cerebral death may never develop, but the patient may die as the result of the failure of other systems, particularly the cardiovascular. Although both cerebral death and irreversible coma usually terminate within a short time in cardiac arrest, their distinction is essential, for cerebral death now has statutory recognition, whereas irreversible coma is only a broad clinical concept.

A third problem relates to the common use of the term "cerebral death" to imply certain pathophysiological states. Thus, the clinician describes it as "a state of irreversible deterioration of nerve tissue so severe that the brain is no longer capable of maintaining 'internal hemostasis' " (378). For the physiologist, "brain death" is the result of an "exclusive intracranial circulatory arrest involving both carotid and vertebral basilar systems" (22) and producing a "total brain infarction." The electroencephalographer (11) views brain death as present when a patient "not under the influence of sedative drug intoxication, hypothermia or deep anesthesia, satisfies all clinical and electroencephalographic criteria for brain death for some length of time." Then, in line with the more social aspects of medicine, some doctors have expressed a growing feeling that brain death may be present when the individual, although capable of some vital functions such as respiration and cardiovascular control, has lost the capability of reacting to external stimuli and remains in an unresponsive vegetative state (477).

These various connotations associated with the term cerebral death are confusing to both the physician and the layman. For this reason, to denote a dead brain in a living body by a new name free of encumbering attributes is desirable. Orthothanasia has been used with the meaning of deliberately ending artificial or heroic means of maintaining life. Encephalothanasia, the direct Greek translation of the term used in many languages for cerebral death, although somewhat long, would seem to be appropriate, and, being new, to have none of the linguistic misconnotations of the older term.

Abbreviations

The following abbreviations are used in the text:

BA . . . . biological activity
CBF . . . . cerebral blood flow
CD . . . . cerebral death
CNS . . . . central nervous system
ECS . . . . electrocerebral silence
EEG . . . . . electroencephalogram or electroencephalography
EKG . . . . .electrocardiogram
EMG . . . . electromyogram
ICP . . . . intracranial pressure
rCBF . . . . regional cerebral blood flow
SAH . . . . subarachnoid hemorrhage
SAP . . . . systemic arterial pressure

Chapter II

Epidemiology of Cerebral Death

Introduction

Cerebral death is an iatrogenic state resulting from the advances in re-suscitative techniques. Consequently, it occurs more frequently in large medical institutions with active emergency rooms and large neurology and neurosurgical services. Even under such conditions, its incidence is approximately 1% of all deaths, so that it is not a common state.

The Collaborative Study Plan

Information concerning the epidemiology of cerebral death may be derived from the results of the Collaborative Study (99).

Protocol. This study was designed to identify criteria that might characterize persons with a dead brain. Accordingly, the requirements for admission to the study had to be broad enough to encompass all individuals in danger of imminent death and yet be sufficiently restrictive to exclude most people with reversible brain damage. Cerebral unresponsivity and apnea were selected as basic criteria for admission to this study upon the

9

assumption that they indicated lack of cerebral hemispheral and brainstem function respectively. *Cerebral unresponsivity* was defined as a state in which the patient did not respond purposely to externally applied stimuli, obeyed no commands, and did not phonate spontaneously or in response to painful stimuli. *Apnea* was arbitrarily defined as neurogenic impairment of breathing requiring a respirator for a period of at least 15 minutes.

The protocol for the collaborative program required that all patients over the age of one year who were admitted to one of nine participating hospitals in a comatose and apneic state lasting for 15 minutes, or who developed such a condition in the course of hospitalization, were to be seen immediately by a member of the study team. If the patient did not meet the above criteria, the team followed him or her at 12-hour intervals until the criteria were met or the patient recovered or died.

Upon a patient's entry into the study, a concise history, neurological examination, provisional diagnosis, status of the vital signs, physical findings, medications and therapeutic procedures were documented. Blood was drawn for screening for drugs, especially barbiturates. An electroencephalogram using standard montages and under approved recording conditions was made as soon after the neurological examination as possible. Certain additional laboratory determinations required for treatment of the patient were usually obtained; these included urinalysis (with measurement of daily fluids, input and output), blood counts, blood chemistries, blood gases and cerebrospinal fluid analyses.

The patient was then followed at 6, 12, and 24 hours by neurological and EEG examinations. If the patient had electrocerebral silence (ECS) for 24 hours, the attending physician had the prerogative to discontinue all resuscitative efforts or to follow the patient with daily neurological and EEG examinations until the heart stopped beating. After the 24 hours, if ECS was not present, the patient was reexamined daily, both neurologically and electroencephalographically, for 3 days and then twice a week until ECS, improvement or cardiac arrest occurred. Upon the development of ECS, the patient was placed on the daily examination routine. Patients improving were followed for 3 months or until a decision to withdraw the patient from the study was made by the family or personal physician.

Admission to the study did not interfere with the routine medical care of the patient. The investigators observed and recorded results of the various tests, but the patient's right to "death with dignity" as prescribed by the personal physician and the family was never compromised by the activities of the cerebral survival program.

The data on the 503 patients studied in all the centers were pooled and analyzed as a unit. This statistical treatment of the material tends to eliminate some of the inherent peculiarities of the population of certain centers.

Population at Risk

Although many conditions may result in a dead brain, there are certain afflictions that have a predilection to neurological complications ending in cerebral death. In a general hospital population, the most common causes of coma and apnea—the hallmarks of a dead brain—are cerebrovascular, cardiac and traumatic disorders, the three accounting for more than two-thirds of all cases entered in the Collaborative Study (Table II–1). The long list of other etiologies includes many of the disorders to which humanity is subject. In a great number of these conditions, cardiovascular or pulmonary disturbances contributed to or precipitated coma and apnea. Obviously, the population referred to any given hospital will determine the relative proportions of the disease entities that produce a dead brain. For this reason, other writers have reported quite different proportions of conditions giving rise to coma and apnea. Plum and Posner, (378) for example, have few cases of cardiac arrest in their series, while neurosurgical centers have a disproportionately large number of persons with head injuries and brain tumors.

Age and Sex. In the age distribution, the presence of two peaks, one in the teens and one in the fifties, presumably reflects the human age predilection for traumatic and vascular disorders respectively. The fact that males predominate (Table II–2) undoubtedly relates to the greater risk in men to conditions producing deep coma, such as cerebral trauma and cardiac infarction.

Table II–1.   Primary Diagnosis in Collaborative Study.

Admission Diagnosis	Total Number of Cases
Cardiac disorders (mainly infarction)	105
Cerebral trauma	94
Cerebral thrombosis	25
Subarachnoid hemorrhage	34
Cerebral embolism	8
Cerebral hemorrhage	74
Cerebral (other)	9
Central nervous system infection	17
Exogenous intoxication	36
Metabolic disorder	36
Neoplasm	12
Other	53
Total	503

Table II–2.   Age and Sex of Population in Collaborative Study.

Age (by decade)	Sex		Total
	Female	Male	
<10	25	18	43
10–19	27	31	58
20–29	19	29	48
30–39	18	26	44
40–49	34	39	73
50–59	44	47	91
60–69	30	50	80
70–79	23	28	51
>80	8	7	15
Totals	228	275	503

Table II–3.   Elapsed Time From Cerebral Insult to Cerebral Unresponsiveness and Apnea.

Elapsed Time	Number of Cases	
	Insult to Unresponsiveness	Insult to Apnea
<1.9 hours	333	219
2–3.9 hours	22	34
4–7.9 hours	13	44
8–15.9 hours	10	33
16 hours to 2 days	34	59
>2 days	58	83
Unknown	33	31
Total	503	503

The Natural History of Deep Coma and Cerebral Death.   In most cases, the onset of the cerebral insult was abrupt, and coincided with coma. However, unresponsiveness might be delayed several days after the cerebral insult (Table II–3). Similarly, the time between the ictus and respiratory arrest varied, although in many cases they were noted simultaneously. Artificial ventilation was usually started before, at the time of, or shortly after respiratory arrest. The resuscitative efforts unquestionably influenced the course of the disorder. Their early application improved the outcome, for in one center in which treatment was started soon after the ictus the mortality was 69.1% as compared to 84.4% for the other centers. In these severely brain-injured patients, the effect of medications seems to have been minimal. In fact, although the differences are slight, the patients not receiving medications (probably the less seriously injured) in all instances did better than those pharmacologically treated (Table II–4).

Table II–4.   Relationship of Initial Medications* and Therapeutic Procedures Prescribed to Outcome (503 Cases).

	Prescribed	(% Survivors)	Not Prescribed	(% Survivors)
Medication				
Analgesics, sedatives or				
tranquilizers	150	(6)	353	(9)
Antibiotic agents	145	(4)	358	(10)
Blood substitutes	29	(3)	474	(8)
Cortico-steroids	233	(5)	270	(11)
Vasopressors	98	(3)	405	(9)
Other drugs	332	(6)	171	(12)
Therapeutic Procedure				
Craniotomy	5	(20)	498	(8)
Dialysis	16	(12)	487	(8)
Hypothermia	54	(2)	449	(9)
Other or none	446	(9)	57	(6)

*Many patients had multiple drugs.

Only two therapeutic procedures were used commonly in patients of this study (Table II–4). Dialysis, as therapy for intoxications, was effectively employed in almost half of the drug cases. Its effect on the pathological picture in those cases that succumbed is difficult to determine because there were few such cases, all complicated by factors other than intoxication. Hypothermia, which theoretically might have benefited coma due to cerebral infarction, was rarely used energetically in this series. The lowest temperature recorded in the 2,280 rectal readings made was 78° F, and only 45 readings (2%) were under 90° F. These temperature did not seem either to protect the brain or make it more susceptible to pathological changes.

Fate of Persons Meeting Entrance Criteria.   The outcome of the 503 cases admitted to the study is given in Table II–5. Although 50 patients were discharged alive, 6 of these died within the arbitrary three-month limit of the study. Thus, of the cases admitted on the basis of coma and apnea, more than 90% died.

The time of death (Table II–6) measured from entrance to the study peaks at one to two days, probably, in part, owing to the discontinuance at that time of resuscitative measures on cases suspected of cerebral death. But even if the patients on whom resuscitation was stopped are excluded, the peak is still at 1 to 1.9 days. Some patients lingered for more than a month before death occurred.

Of the 50 patients who survived for sufficient time to be discharged from the study, six died of their primary disorder within three months. Three additional patients who had made a satisfactory recovery from drug in-

Table II–5.   Final Disposition of Cases.

Disposition	Total Number of Cases
Cardiac death	345
Cerebral death[1]	114
Recovery, complete[2]	26
Recovery, incomplete[3]	15
Recovery, degree unknown[4]	3
Total	503

[1] Cases in which resuscitation was stopped, presumably on the basis of cerebral death
[2] 23 drug intoxication, 2 cardiac disease and 1 stroke
[3] 4 cerebral trauma, 3 cardiac, 1 each drug intoxication, cerebrovascular disease, metabolic disease and brain tumor and 4 other
[4] 3 drug intoxication

Table II–6.   Time of Death from Entrance to Study.

Elapsed Time	Total Cases	Resuscitation Stopped*
<1 hour	4	0
1–5.9	51	6
6–11.9	33	5
12–23.9	63	16
1–1.9 days	143	68
2–2.9	54	11
3–3.9	33	4
4–6.9	35	2
1–1.9 weeks	21	1
2–3.9	13	1
4	9	0
Total dead	459	114

*Patients on whom resuscitative measures were discontinuned by the attending physician, presumably on the basis of a diagnosis of cerebral death.

toxication failed to report for followup, so their statuses are unknown. There remain 41 persons who were alive for at least three months after admission to the study. Of these survivors, 24 had a primary diagnosis of drug intoxication, and an additional 4 were known to have exogenous intoxications complicating another primary disorder. All but one of the uncomplicated drug cases recovered completely. The degree of recovery in the other cases, with the exception of one transient stroke and two cardiac cases whose cerebral statuses were completely restored, was considered incomplete. One patient was able to follow a useful life, but the remainder had dependent existences, and one of these died about four months after entry into the study.

Differential Diagnosis

The conditions that may simulate cerebral death are many; in fact, any of the numerous causes of coma may produce a state resembling that of a dead brain. However, in most comatose conditions, respiration is preserved, at least, until cardiac arrest is imminent. The deliriums, dementias and hypersomnias all retain respiration even when there is no response to any form of stimulation. The neurological states resulting from upper brainstem lesions—persistent vegetative state, akinetic mutism, apallic syndrome, locked-in-state, etc.—are likewise associated with spontaneous breathing, although occasionally in the early acute phase some respiratory alterations are present.

The term "apallic syndrome" has been advocated as a designation for the clinical state of complete loss of higher functions such as speech, voluntary motor activity, emotional reactions, but with retention of brainstem function. Originally, the term was introduced by Kretchmer to denote clinical states resulting from loss of the pallium, the gray cortical mantle. Subsequent writers used the term somewhat loosely to include transient comatose states such as might follow cerebral trauma. In the English literature these conditions were referred to as prolonged unconsciousness, persistent vegetative state or decorticate or decerebrate states. The French introduced such terms as coma prolongé, or coma vigilé. These patients may live for months or sometimes years. Ingvar (204) cites two patients who survived 8 and 17 years in a comatose, poorly responsive state. On neuropathological examination a massive necrosis of the gray matter was found with involvement of the basal ganglia and in some cases the thalamus. In addition, the cerebellar Purkinje cells were in some cases practically wiped out, and brainstem neurons had some degeneration. Regional blood flow studies in some of Ingvar's cases showed impaired blood flow in the cerebral hemispheres but high rates over the basal parts corresponding to the brainstem. Clinically these patients were deeply comatose after their initial episode, which, in most cases, was a cerebral anoxia, but within a few days, spontaneous respiration, brainstem and some cranial nerve reflexes returned. Thermal, electrolyte and water regulation were preserved. These patients could be aroused, exhibited primitive avoidance movements, could chew and had respiratory alterations on irritation. Electroencephalographically, some showed paroxysmal discharges, but in most cases, the electroencephalogram was depressed or even isoelectric with no evoked potentials.

There are a few conditions simulating cerebral death in which respiration may be in abeyance, namely, drug intoxication, deep hypothermia and polyneuritis. The most common cause of drug intoxication is one of the barbiturates, but the various pep or trip pills are often responsible. Opiates may be the causative agent, especially in drug addicts. Other drugs, such as the muscle paralyzers (curare, etc.) may produce a locked-in syndrome that, unless suspected, may be difficult to diagnose. Since some of these drugs depress the cortical potentials, the electroencephalogram may be isoelectric. Blood analyses may give nontoxic levels of the drug even though the individual is comatose. This is particularly true if multiple drugs, especially alcohol, have been ingested. The latter has synergistic effects with many drugs, so that even small amounts may cause a deep coma.

Metabolic disorders are a common cause of coma, but rarely is respiration abolished in the early stages.

A hypothermic state is likely to develop in chronically debilitated or alcoholic individuals, especially if they are exposed to the cold. At temperatures below 30° C, the cerebral and body metabolism is so lowered that respiration may be imperceptible and the patient may lapse into coma. This hypothermic state has been mistaken for death; in fact, most of the examples of persons being buried alive in the past century were the result of such exposure. It was upon rewarming in a coffin or morgue that these Lazaruses were resurrected. The body temperature may drop as the result of a dead brain, but rarely to such low levels (Table III–2). If the temperature is below 35° C, the individual should be rewarmed before tests for cerebral death are applied.

On rare occasions, a generalized polyneuritis, occasionally of the Guillain-Barré type, will produce a complete paralysis of all muscles so that the person, although alert, cannot communicate. If the patient was not seen in the early stages when speech was still possible, the condition may be difficult to diagnose. However, pupillary reactions are often still present and the EEG is normal. Years ago, before cerebral death was recognized, poliomyelitis occasionally presented such a locked-in syndrome.

Posner (380) emphasizes that a number of conditions may simulate aspects of a dead brain. Various drugs will give rise to fixation of the pupils. Certain vestibular depressants may abolish oculovestibular reflexes. Neuromuscular blockers may produce a lack of motor activity. An isoelectric electroencephalogram may be caused by sedative drugs, hypothermia, encephalitis, trauma and even arterial hypotension. The various causes of impaired consciousness must also be considered. However, with all this in mind, a careful neurological examination, supplemented by laboratory and radiological examinations, will enable a diagnosis to be established.

Chapter III

Clinical Findings in Cerebral Death

Introduction

The clinical aspects of acute death are well known, but the manifestations of death in comatose patients maintained by life-support measures are not so well established nor so easily recognized. Asgian et al. (26) recorded electromyograms (EMG), electrocardiograms (EKG), electroencephalograms (EEG) and pneumograms as patients, comatose as the result of cerebrovascular disease, passed into death. In the premortal stage, myoclonic jerking of the chin and ocular muscles and transient respiratory and EKG changes were noted. The EEG had less activity on the diseased side, but respiratory, muscular and movement artifacts were present bilaterally at the moment of clinical death, as contrasted to the flat records of the EKG and pneumogram. After a few minutes, the EEG traces also became isoelectric, first over the diseased hemisphere and then on the normal side. When a deeper coma with imperceptible EEG activity was present, cardiac death was manifested by a slowing of the usually abnormal EKG until ventricular contractions stopped altogether. Korein (251) has also shown the varied EKG changes that occur as the myocardium ceases its contractions.

The sequence of events as cerebral death ensues has been described by Gaches et al. (141). Decerebration almost always occurred (in 69 of 71 cases) before apnea, and was followed by areflexia and hypotonia. Then mydriasis usually developed, succeeded by arterial hypotension and, 3–4 hours later, hypothermia. The electroencephalogram became flat some hours after apnea, at about the same time as cerebral circulatory collapse.

Since brain death is the irreversible cessation of cerebral function, its basic characteristics are often described under the headings of cerebral activity, vital functions and cephalic reflexes, all of which must be absent to establish cerebral death.

Cerebral Responsivity

Cerebral activity involves high level faculties such as perception, voluntary movement, ideation, memory, etc., that underlie the general state of awareness referred to as consciousness. Since individual higher mental functions may be impaired and even lost by localized brain lesions, the identification of a dead brain requires not just impaired consciousness but the total absence of awareness—i.e., a deep coma.

Coma (Cerebral unresponsivity).   Coma may be due to widespread cortical or subcortical lesions, or it may be the result of damage to the brainstem. In cerebral death, there is total unawareness of external or internal excitation, so that even the most painful stimuli evoke neither vocal nor purposeful response. Although this statement lacks scientific precision, there is no difficulty in clinical practice in recognizing the condition; defense or other spinal reflexes rarely are responsible for movements that are confused with cerebrally induced and purposeful responses.

Vital Functions

The lack of control of the vital functions—temperature, pulse, and respiration—has naturally been considered as a cardinal manifestation of cerebral death. Certainly, respiration is completely abolished in patients suspected of having brain death. However, the impairment of the other vital signs related to temperature control and cardiac function is less obligatory.

Apnea.   Neurosurgeons have long noted that respiratory arrest resulted from encroachment upon the brainstem by transtentorial herniations, or from pressure on the medulla oblongata due to cerebellar tonsillar coning into the foramen magnum. It is not surprising, then, that apnea is an early indication of impending cerebral death, usually present before signs of cardiovascular involvement appear. Manual artificial respiration is commonly used until more appropriate methods of pulmonary ventilation can be applied. Although breathing may only require assistance initially, respiration usually becomes entirely dependent upon mechanical ventilation within a short time. When cerebral death is suspected, many authors, as a check on spontaneous respiration, have recommended stopping artificial respiration for various periods of time. The Harvard criteria state "the total absence of spontaneous breathing may be established by turning off the respirator for three minutes and observing whether there is any effort on the part of the subject to breathe spontaneously . . . provided that at the start of the trial period the patient's carbon dioxide tension is within the normal range, and provided also that the patient has been breathing room air for at least 10 minutes prior to the trial" (34). Similar but usually less specific requirements have been made by other authors. According to Plum and Posner, "if the PCO_2 is within normal range and the patient had been breathing room air for 10 minutes prior to the trial, 1 or 2 minutes without artificial respiration should produce a CO_2 tension high enough to near-maximally stimulate the respiratory centers. If blood gas determinations are not easily available, the respiratory function may be tested by the technique of apneic oxygenation . . . (in which) the patient is respired with 100% oxygen for 10 to 20 minutes and then the respirator is disconnected and oxygen delivered through a catheter to the trachea at the rate of 6 liters per minute . . . This allows PCO_2 to rise without any danger of further hypoxia, and the apneic patient may be safely observed for periods of 7 to 10 minutes" (378).

The Royal Colleges and Faculties of the United Kingdom (399) give even more specific directions for checking on the permanency of apnea. During this test it is necessary for the arterial carbon dioxide tension ($PaCO_2$) to exceed the threshold for respiratory stimulation—that is, the $PaCO_2$ should normally reach 50 mm Hg (6.65 kPa). This is best achieved by measurement of the blood gases; if this facility is available it is recommended that the patient should be disconnected when the $PaCO_2$ reaches 40–45 mm Hg following administration of 5% CO_2 in oxygen through the ventilator. This starting level has been chosen because patients may be moderately hypothermic (35–37° C), flaccid and have a depressed metabolic rate, so that arterial carbon-dioxide tension rises only slowly in apnea (about 2 mm Hg/min). (Hypoxia during disconnection should be prevented by delivering oxygen at 6 liters/min through a catheter into the trachea.) If blood-gas analysis is not available to measure the $PaCO_2$, the alternative procedure is to supply the ventilator with pure oxygen for ten minutes (pre-oxygenation), then with 5% CO_2 in oxygen for five minutes, and to disconnect the ventilator for ten minutes while delivering oxygen at 6 liters/min by catheter into the trachea (399). However, no precise data have been given regarding the effect of this practice on blood gases, pH or electrolytes.

The reliability and safety of such trials has been questioned. Pilot studies showed that the arterial oxygen pressure PaO_2 would have to fall to dangerously low levels and the venous CO_2 pressure ($PvCO_2$) rise to levels potentially toxic to diseased organs before stimulating respiration. Accordingly, the Collaborative Study concluded that a three-minute test off the respirator would be inadequate and inadvisable. As an entrance criterion, apnea was considered established if a person showed no evidence of spontaneous respiration and required artificial ventilation for at least 15 minutes. If spontaneous respiratory efforts occur at the bedside, bucking the intratracheal tube is readily recognized.

However, for the pronouncement of cerebral death, more definitive means of certifying permanent apnea were necessary. For that purpose, after all other clinical and electroencephalographic criteria had been met, as a final test, the patient was taken off the respirator and watched for respiratory efforts. Rarely was there any attempt to breathe spontaneously, and if gasps occurred, they were insufficient to maintain respiration.

Subsequent studies indicated that this procedure was inadequate to raise the $PvCO_2$ to levels sufficient to stimulate the normal respiratory center, and yet it depleted the PaO_2 to dangerously low levels (Table III–1).

The problem was studied in detail by Milhaud et al. (317, 318). They noted return of respiration in three comatose and apneic patients after more than 5 minutes off the ventilator. Moreover, they encountered complications as the result of the hypoxia. For these reasons, they discontinued this test. However, they believed that transient hyperapnia without hypoxia would not harm even diseased hearts or brains. They concluded that a safe and simple test is to administer 100% oxygen for more than one hour to de-nitrogenize the blood before discontinuing the respirator. If a small catheter is then introduced into the endotracheal tube and oxygen administered at the rate of 4 to 5 liters per minute, the PaO_2 will be approximately

Table III–1.   Blood Gases After Cessation of Respiration (*courtesy of Dr. P. Turner*).

Time (min.)	pH	PCO$_2$	PO$_2$	Bicarb	O$_2$ Sat
0*	7.55	16	39	14	82
3	7.47	18	30	13	63
6	7.48	13	21	10	41
9	7.45	20	15	14	<40

*Patient was artificially breathing 40% O_2 until this time.

300 mm Hg (if it is not above 100 mm Hg, the test should not be done) and even after 20 minutes of apnea will not fall below 250 mm Hg. At the same time, if the patient is normothermic, the $PaCO_2$ rises to levels much above the threshold of normal excitation of the respiratory center (50–60 mm Hg). However, Caronna, in a discussion of Milhaud et al.'s paper (318, p. 264), pointed out that as a high $PaCO_2$ depresses respiration and a pH below 7.0 depresses brain function, it would be advisable not to exceed a $PaCO_2$ of 60, which gives maximal stimulation to the respiratory center. This is particularly pertinent as many patients suspected of cerebral death already have damaged organs (infarcted hearts), which may be unusually susceptible to hypercarbia or acidosis.

In practice, Milhaud et al. (318) take arterial blood every 3 minutes after the denitrogenization for blood gases to confirm that the PaO_2 is above 100 mm Hg and that $PaCO_2$ reaches a level of 60 mm Hg. Under these conditions the absence of spontaneous respiration after 15 minutes is evidence of permanent apnea.

On the basis of extensive clinical experience, Pitts et al. (375), although, at first, doubting that a $PaCO_2$ of 50-60 mm Hg was adequate to stimulate the medullary respiratory, eventually confirmed the conclusions of the French writers (318, p. 264).

Rectal Temperature.   An inability to regulate temperature—a poikilothermic state—is often cited as an indication of cerebral death. However, Lausberg (274) pointed out that hypothermia is not synonymous with loss of temperature regulation. He considered temperatures as low as 34° C as reversible. Schneider (410) thinks that the impaired thermoregulation in cerebral death resembles the reversible hypothermia that accompanies the spinal shock seen in high cervical cord lesions. Indeed, the analogy appears appropriate, for in cerebral death the spinomedullary junction is the site of severe myelopathy. Lausberg (274) points out that damage at the midbrain level, manifested clinically by decerebration, is associated with a disturbance in regulation of heat stress, while adjustment to cold is usually maintained. Injuries at the bulbopontine level may lead to a poikilothermic state with temperatures falling spontaneously below 32° C. Warming will raise the core temperature which again falls when the source of heat is removed. Thermoregulation returns in three weeks after high cervical lesions in experimental animals (275).

Few cerebral death patients have temperatures below 90° F even a few hours before death. There is a tendency, however, for the initial body temperature to be a few degrees higher than the final temperature.

The fear that a poikilothermic state may be associated with body temperatures low enough to produce electrocerebral silence seems unwarranted in clinical practice. In man, it requires a temperature below 29° C to slow the frequency of the EEG potentials: in the dog, the EEG does not become isoelectric until the core temperature reaches 17° C, the level at which vasomotor control fails and the blood pressure falls. In the Collaborative Study, only 12 of 503 patients had temperatures below 90° F; all of these were warmed by external heat to temperatures within the normal range (with the exception of two patients whose temperatures continued to fall as they died). Of these 12 patients, 7 had biological activity (BA) in their EEGs, 5 had electrocerebral silence (ECS) and none had an equivocal (Equiv) record—approximately the same proportion as in the entire series (Table III–2).

The inclusion of hypothermia as a criterion of cerebral death would seem inappropriate (12) on the basis of the above considerations. Moreover, children, by reason of the large ratio of body surface to body volume, and alcoholic patients (whose cutaneous vessels are dilated) may become hypothermic after mild neural injuries. Jährig (214) concluded that although the temperatures of neonates were often low, this was not a reliable sign of cerebral death.

Blood Pressure.   The presence of an unstable blood pressure has been advocated as a criterion of cerebral death. In fact, a Japanese study (469) has made this one of its major criteria for death. This might be a more potent determinant or predictor of death were it not for the fact that patients are ordinarily treated for hypotension by intravenous saline and vasopressor drugs to maintain blood pressure within a normal range. In the Collaborative Study, only about 25% of the patients required vasopressor agents to maintain their pressure and less than 20% had systolic blood pressures below 70 mm Hg at the time of their final clinical examination (Table III–3). When hemodynamic disturbances were present, Yamada et al. (519) found that only noradrenaline was effective in maintaining blood pressure. Isoproterenol had little effect on the ventricular

Table III–2.   Relationship of Initial EEG Findings to Initial Rectal Temperature (Collaborative Study).

Rectal Temperature	EEG Results			
	No.	ECS	Equiv.	BA
Unknown	7	3	1	2
<89.9.....................	12	5	0	7
90– 94.9	55	31	3	20
95– 99.9	265	100	13	138
100–104.9	156	35	11	105
>105	8	1	1	6
Total	503	175	29	278

Table III-3.   Systolic Blood Pressure Initial and Final Examinations (Collaborative Study).

Systolic Pressure	Number of Cases	
	Initial*	Final*
<50	45	78
50–69	38	47
70–89	103	100
90–109	125	119
110–129	84	94
130–149	47	30
150–169	28	20
170–189	15	10
190–209	5	2
>210	13	3
Total	503	503

*Difference is significant at $p < 0.001$

output, blood pressure or venous return curve. Hence, both cardiac and peripheral circulatory mechanisms are severely impaired or abolished in cerebral death. However, since hypopiesia is associated with a low cerebral perfusion pressure, which in turn may abolish EEG activity. Ishiguro et al.'s (210) warning is appropriate: cerebrospinal or spinal shock with cessation of spontaneous movements, atonic musculature and an abrupt fall of blood pressure may be mistaken for brain death.

Pulse Pressure. The pulse pressure does not seem to be a good predictor of cerebral death, for it changes relatively little from the initial to the final examination. Perhaps the large number of patients with pulse pressures greater than 80 mm Hg may indicate the presence of relaxed vascular beds.

Pulse Rate. The frequency of heart beat does not correlate with cerebral death. On the initial examinations in the Collaborative Study, few patients had pulse rates outside of the normal range. In approximately 5% of cases, on the final examination the pulse rate had decreased slightly but not to a very significant degree. It is true that for a few minutes before cardiac death there is a slowing of the pulse rate. Wertheimer et al. (510), in their original description of cerebral death, described several tests for bulbar activity based upon the pulse rate. Sinocarotid and oculocardiac reflexes were examined, but even in normal individuals these reflexes do not constantly cause a perceptible cardiac slowing. Wertheimer et al. also recommended the injection of atropine (1 mg), which acts centrally to accelerate the heart rate. Subsequent writers paid little attention to this test, but recently Lorenz (296) and Ouaknine et al. (359) have confirmed its value as a determinant of medullary activity. In 75 cerebrally dead patients,

Ouaknine found that administration of atropine caused no change in heart rate.

In conclusion: Of the vital signs, only respiratory failure and the absence of a response to intravenous injection of atropine appear to discriminate the inert from the functioning brainstem.

Possibility of Return of Vital Functions. After 15 minutes absence of spontaneous respiration and consciousness, what is the possibility of these functions returning? Granted that many factors, including etiology, time before initiation of treatment, type of treatment, etc., influence the likelihood of restitution of these activities, it may still be instructive to examine the actual data in the Collaborative Study series. Of 431 patients who had multiple examinations, 132 at some time had at least temporary return of respiratory function. Forty-eight recovered within 24 hours, and 2 others at 36 and 49 hours; all 50 were discharged breathing spontaneously. Of the others, 25 had a transient return of respiration at the time of admission to the study, but subsequently died. Another 45 had evidence of respiratory effort in the next 24 hours, but all subsequently succumbed.

Return of responsiveness was less common, only 62 responding after a period of coma. Of these, 50 recovered and 12 subsequently died before discharge from the hospital.

The Cephalic Reflexes

The reflexes mediated by the cranial nerves are important indicators of the integrity of the brainstem. Thus, their absence is an essential part of the brain death syndrome. Just as in clinical neurology, where they have varying significance in diagnosis, so in the identification of a dead brain the individual cephalic reflexes differ in their importance as a criterion of death. Obviously the presence of an intratracheal tube compromises cough and pharyngeal reflexes. Other cranial nerve reflexes may be impaired by local edema or drying of tissues. For these reasons, at times some of the cranial nerve reflexes cannot be adequately tested (Table III–4), and their responses may require critical evaluation. Moreover, more intense stimulation than used in the clinic is needed, since the reflex circuits, if active, are profoundly depressed. Finally, the examination must be done without the cooperation of the patient. Because of these difficulties, some authors have chosen as criteria of cerebral death those cephalic reflexes that they consider to be the most sensitive and discriminative of brainstem function and omitted the other tests that are more difficult to perform and interpret.

Table III–4.   Cephalic Reflexes Untested on Initial Examination (Collaborative Study, 503 Cases).

Reflex	Number of patients untested
Pupillary light	2
Corneal	2
Oculocephalic	8
Audio-ocular	12
Snout	15
Jaw Jerk	24
Vestibular	44
Cough	72
Pharyngeal	79
Swallowing	85

Table III–5.   Correlation of Absence of Cephalic Reflexes on Initial Examination in Comatose and Apneic Patients with Outcome (Collaborative Study).

Reflex	Correlation Coefficient*
	Death
All cephalic	0.2279
Pupillary	0.2787
Corneal	0.1828
Oculocephalic	0.0820
Vestibular	0.1369
Swallowing	0.0726
Jaw jerk	0.0113
Pharyngeal	0.0656
Cough	0.0791
Snout	0.0691
Audio-ocular	0.0310
All spinal	0.1512

*based on Kendall's method (239)

There is justification for this viewpoint since, as will be pointed out, some reflexes are much less discriminative of cerebral death than others (Table III–5).

Allen et al. (9), who have made the most detailed study of the cephalic reflexes in brain death, have noted the wide range of correlations with brain death and survival or cardiac death.

Pupillary Reflex.   The pupillary reflex is classically evoked by flashing a bright light into first one and then the other eye and noting a constriction of the pupil of the eye stimulated (direct response) and a constriction of the other pupil (consensual response). When the pupils are dilated, a constriction is easily observed, but if the pupils are small (2–3 mm) the reaction may be difficult to see. This reflex is perhaps the simplest to elicit and one of the most discriminant of the cephalic reflexes. It tends to return early if recovery is to occur, but may come and go in the process of dying (Fig. III–1).

In the Collaborative Study series, a pupillary reaction was present in 25% of cases and correlated with a 21% chance of survival, as compared with a 4% survival in cases with a nonreacting pupil. In patients with electrocerebral silence, the pupillary reactions were absent in 98.4% of cases (Table III–6).

Although not strictly a reflex, the size of the pupils, which is regulated by the balance of pupilloconstrictor (parasympathetic) and pupillodilator (sympathetic) activities, is an important diagnostic factor. Since transtentorial herniations distort and compress the oculomotor nerves, under such circumstances the pupils tend to be dilated and fixed, whereas pontomedullary lesions that interrupt the sympathetic pathways but leave intact the oculomotor nerves tend to be associated with small pupils.

Although it is commonly stated that the pupils are dilated in cerebral death, a number of authors have pointed out that small or medium-sized pupils are frequently present. Prochazka (386) and his associates (387) have emphasized that mydriasis is not essential for the diagnosis of brain death. In fact, in the Collaborative Study only about half of the patients with other evidence of cerebral death, including ECS, had pupils more than 5 mm in diameter on their initial examination and few dilated as death approached (Table III–7). The size of the pupils was significant in predicting outcome, for twice as many persons with small as with large pupils survived (Table III–7). The pupillary size has added significance because most sedative and narcotic agents are associated with constricted pupils. Thus, in a comatose, apneic person, the presence of small pupils would suggest a dormant brain. Two drugs do produce dilated pupils— glutethimide (doriden®) and scopolamine. The coma of the former may be broken through by repetitive noxious stimulation with return of deep coma upon cessation of the irritation; mydriasis is not a constant feature. Scopolamine and associated anticholinergic drugs tend to produce a severe delirium rather than a stuporous state, associated with signs of parasympathetic dysfunction such as cutaneous vasodilation.

Corneal reflex.   The corneal reflex is usually tested by drawing a wisp of cotton over the cornea and noting a blink response of both eyes. Since this unilateral corneal stimulation induces a bilateral closure of the eyelids, the response, if present, is readily observed. However, edema or drying of the cornea may prevent an adequate stimulus and thus abolish the response. It is absent in practically all cases of ECS, and returns early if

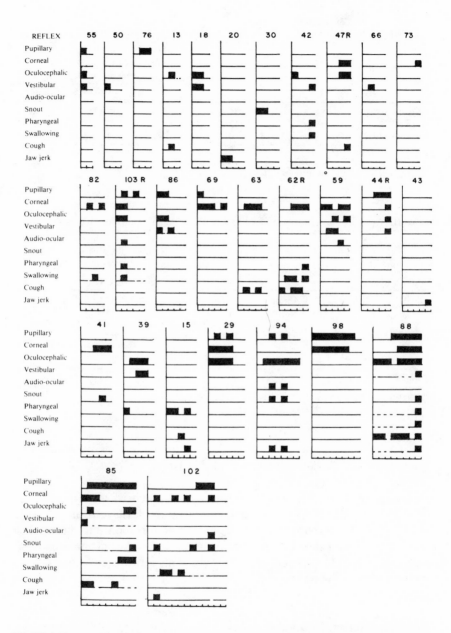

Fig. III–1. Bar graphs to indicate the status of the cephalic reflexes in those cases that showed changes after the initial insult in a series of 100 comatose and apneic patients. The numbers refer to the case designation; an appended "R" indicates recovery. The interval between spikes on the line at the base indicates the time of examination—0, 6, 12, 24, 48, 72 hours and every third day. A line opposite the reflex at the time interval represents absence of the reflex, a black box the presence of the reflex, and an interrupted line denotes no examination reported.

Table III–6.   Relationship of Pupillary Reactions to EEG Findings (Collaborative Study).

| Pupillary Reaction | Initial EEG Findings Number of Cases (percentage of survivors in brackets) | | | |
	BA	Equivocal	ECS	Total
Absent*	171 (8)	28	183 (1)	382 (4)
Present*	112 (21)	1	3	116 (21)
Other or unknown	0	1	1	2
Totals	283	30	187	500

*Difference is significant at p<0.001

Table III–7.   Relationship of Size of Pupils to EEG Findings (Collaborative Study).

| Size of Pupils | Initial EEG Findings Number of Cases (percentage of survivors in brackets) | | | |
	BA	Equivocal	ECS	Total
Equal ....1–4 mm*	29 (70)	8	142 (2)	179 (13)
5–8 mm*	104 (12)	14	75	193 (6)
<8	4	—	3	7
Unequal both ....<5 mm	11 (36)	2	23	36 (11)
. >5 mm	22 (5)	3	12	37 (3)
Other or unknown	17 (5)	3	28	48 (2)
Totals	187 (22)	30	283 (1)	500

*Difference is significant at p<0.001

the patient shows signs of survival (unless the cornea has become insensitive due to edema or dehydration (Table III–8).

Oculocephalic Reflex (Doll's eyes response).   Upon brisk movement of the head to one side, the eyes normally conjugately deviate to the opposite side, but remain looking straight ahead when the response is absent. The reflex is mediated through arcs involving the vestibular mechanisms, medial longitudinal bundle and ocular nerves. This reflex is easy to elicit and interpret. It is quite discriminative, and with evidence of recovery it returns early.

Vestibular Reflex.   Provided the external auditory foramen and tympanic membrane are intact, the vestibular reflex is elicited by elevating the head 30° above the horizontal, inserting a small catheter in the canal to the tympanic membrane and slowly injecting 10 cc of ice water. A response is a slow ipsiversive movement of the eyes with or without a fast return component. Responses of the two ears are compared. This reflex is slightly

Table III–8. Cephalic Reflexes at Initial and Final Examinations.

Reflex		Initial (cases)	Final (cases)
All Absent	. . . .	281 (53%)	309 (58.3%)
Pupillary	absent	384	385
	present	117 (23.4%)	112 (22.6%)
	other	2	6
Corneal	absent	411	387
	present	90 (18%)	110 (22.1%)
	other	2	6
Oculocephalic	absent	432	415
	present	63 (12.7%)	71 (14.6%)
	other	8	17
Vestibular	absent	391	374
	present	68 (14.8%)	62 (14.2%)
	other	44	67
Audio-ocular	absent	486	450
	present	5 (1%)	39 (7.9%)
	other	12	14
Snout	absent	465	459
	present	23 (4.7%)	29 (5.9%)
	other	15	15
Pharyngeal	absent	398	384
	present	26 (6.1%)	56 (13%)
	other	79	63
Swallowing	absent	393	379
	present	25 (6%)	63 (14.2%)
	other	85	61
Cough	absent	407	391
	present	24 (5.6%)	55 (12.3%)
	other	72	57
Jaw Jerk	absent	440	441
	present	39 (8.1%)	47 (9.6%)
	other	24	15

more complicated to induce and interpret than the previous ones, and, in practice, it is less commonly examined (Table III–8). However, it is quite discriminative for cerebral death. Upon recovery, it is slightly slower to return than the pupillary and corneal reflexes.

The oculovestibular reflex has been recognized by most investigators as a sensitive and reliable indicator of brainstem function (9, 184, 327, 492). However, as consultants will attest, it is a cranial nerve reflex that is often neglected in the routine neurological examination, even of a comatose patient (99).

Audio-ocular Reflex. The audio-ocular reflex is a blink of the eyelids in response to a sudden clap. Although simple, unfortunately it is not as discriminating as the other cephalic reflexes and is somewhat slower to recover.

Snout Reflex.   A tongue blade is placed over the closed lips and its base is tapped with a percussion hammer. Normally the lips purse. This reflex is simple but it is not particularly discriminative, and sometimes is difficult to obtain in normal individuals.

Pharyngeal (Gag) Reflex.   When the posterior pharynx is touched, the constrictor of the pharynx contracts, producing a gag. The reflex is often compromised by tubes in the throat and dryness of the mucosa, and so the significance of its absence is uncertain (Table III–8).

Swallowing Reflex.   Mucus or water placed on the tongue is swallowed. In the comatose patient, the dehydrated condition of the throat impairs this reflex.

Cough Reflex.   When suction is used in the posterior nasopharynx or trachea, coughing is induced. The reflex is compromised by the intratracheal tube in apneic patients.

Jaw Jerk.   With the thumb upon the chin exerting a slight pressure, tapping the thumb induces contractions of the temporal muscles closing the jaw. This reflex, which is fairly constant in normal people, is moderately discriminative for cerebral death.

A satisfactory examination of the cephalic reflexes is often difficult because of the therapeutic activity. In the Collaborative Study, absence of all cephalic reflexes was noted in more than half of the cases (Table III–8). The individual reflexes varied considerably in their sensitivity to cerebral damage. At the one end, the audio-ocular reflex was abolished in 99% of cases and, at the other end of the scale, the pupillary reflex was absent in only 76.6%. Thus the audio-ocular was extremely sensitive to brain injury and the pupillary only moderately so.

Because clinicians often do not examine all the cranial nerve reflexes, in some sets of criteria for cerebral death certain combinations of reflexes related to the cranial nerves have been specified as essential for the diagnosis of cerebral death. Although, for absolute certainty, all cranial nerve reflexes must be checked, a high degree of certainty may be obtained with certain combinations. Allen et al. (9) have concluded that the most discriminative combination is absence of the pupillary reaction to light, the oculocephalic reflex and the vestibular reflex. However, the degree of probability varies with the time of examination, being somewhat greater at six hours after insult than at the initial examination.

Restoration of Cranial Nerve Function.   Although in comatose and apneic patients, after the initial insult, the status of the individual cranial reflexes generally remains stationary or worsens, in almost 25% of cases one or more reflexes at some time show restitution of function (Table III-9). The corneal, pupillary, oculocephalic and cough reflexes are the most likely to regain responsivity, but any of the cephalic reflexes may be absent on one occasion and be present later. If the patient survives sufficiently long, the cycle may be repeated several times. Usually only 3 or 4 reflexes so fluctuate, not necessary simultaneously, in any one patient. The return of several cephalic reflexes on one or more examinations does not necessarily predict recovery, for death may follow almost as commonly as survival (Figure III-1). Jorgensen (224) noted that individuals with primary brain lesions rarely had a return of cortical activity or cranial nerve reflexes once they were lost, whereas patients comatose as the result of extracranial disorders or drug intoxications regained cortical or brainstem activity often, as the circulatory state improved.

Since the outcome is usually fatal, it would be expected that cephalic reflexes preserved initially might be lost at some subsequent examination. Indeed, of the 29 cases in which the reflexes changed, 17 ultimately had a loss of reflex activity.

Spinal Reflexes

The spinal reflexes, although modulated by cortical and subcortical centers, are basically dependent upon reflex arcs in the spinal cord. For this reason,

Table III–9. The State of the Cephalic Reflexes from Time of Entry to Discharge, 100 Cases

Status		Number of Patients	
No Change			71*
Change			29†
Reflex	Loss	Recovery	Total
Pupillary	4	8	12
Corneal	6	9	15
Oculocephalic	7	8	14
Vestibular	5	6	11
Audio-ocular	0	4	4
Snout	1	5	6
Pharyngeal	2	6	7
Swallowing	0	6	6
Cough	3	7	7
Jaw Jerk	1	5	6
Total cases	17	12	29†

*all died
†25 died; 4 survived

it is understandable that they might persist after cerebral destruction. In fact, if an individual lived long enough for spinal shock to pass off, some spinal reflexes might become hyperactive. Although early writers hypothesized that total areflexia should be present in cerebral death, as experience accumulated it became apparent that spinal reflexes were often present when the brain was dead by all usual criteria.

Tendon Reflexes.   Many writers have noted the preservation of tendon reflexes of the arms and legs in patients otherwise cerebrally dead. Jorgensen et al (227) stated that two thirds of their 42 patients had tendon reflexes. At the initial examination in the Collaborative Study, about half of the patients suspected of cerebral death had absent tendon reflexes in the upper extremity, and almost two thirds were without reflexes in the lower extremity. In subsequent examinations, the state of the tendon reflexes changed little; a few individuals regained their leg reflexes and a few lost their arm reflexes (Table III-10).

Table III–10.   The State of the Spinal Reflexes at Initial and Final Examinations (Collaborative Study).

		Examination (503 cases)	
		Initial	Final
Muscle Tone		325	367
Arm	tone absent	347	381
	tone present	151	115
	other	5	7
Leg	tone absent	342	376
	tone present	159	121
	other	2	6
Superficial Reflex			
All Absent		305	315
Abdominal	absent	461	440
	present	17	31
	other	25	32
Plantar	absent	326	335
	extensor	94	60
	flexor	79	102
	other	4	6
Tendon Reflex			
All Absent		243	247
Arm	absent	267	270
	present	234	227
	other	2	6
Leg	absent	326	309
	present	173	187
	other	4	7

Superficial Reflexes.   Only 3% of individuals suspected of cerebral death have abdominal reflexes on their initial examination, although before death another 3% regain these reflexes. Bronisch (72) reported two cases in which the abdominal reflexes persisted after other evidence, including ECS and cerebral circulatory arrest, indicated a dead brain.

The state of the plantar reflexes in cerebral death is quite different from that of the abdominal reflexes. Although more than 60% of individuals suspected of cerebral death have no plantar responses, those that do have a reflex are slightly more likely to have extensor than flexor responses. However, as time goes on, almost a third of those having extensor responses develop flexor responses, while a few lose their responsivity to plantar stimulation.

Muscle Tone.   The proprioceptive reflexes that control muscle tone and motor activity are severely impaired in cerebral death. In the Collaborative Study, almost 70% of cases had absence of muscle tone in either arms or legs, and 60% in both. Another 10% lost their muscle tone sometime before death.

Motor Activity.   Spontaneous or induced movement may be the result of spinal or cerebral activity. When the brain is undergoing ischemic infarction, the levels of function may be progressively lost so that decorticate, decerebrate and spinal activities appear. In some cases this progress may be followed; Gaches et al. (141) state that decerebrate movements are almost always seen (69 of 71 cases) in the early stages before apnea, and then are lost as the full-blown syndrome of cerebral death develops.

Spontaneous, random movements, usually of the arms, may be seen in patients with all other signs of brain death Allen et al. (9) found that the absence of movements had a weak discriminative coefficient between brain death and other comatose and apneic patients. However, they considered that they should be included as criteria of brain death, since the presence of jerks or spasms, obvious to relatives, might cause concern.

In the Collaborative Study, abnormal posturing was noted in 14% of cases at the initial examination, but in only half that number at the final examination. These movements probably reflect brainstem activity, and it is therefore not surprising that of the 13 cases with posturing on the final examination, only one had a respirator brain. Although more commonly present, less coordinated movements—spasms, jerking, etc.— also tended to disappear. Movements induced by noxious stimuli applied to the extremities or neck represent spinal reflexes which may occur as part of the flexor reflex, although other spinal reflexes—extensor—may occasionally be present. In the upper extremities, extensor reflexes such as those characterizing high spinal cord transections may be induced. Jorgensen (222) emphasized that unilateral pronator and extensor movements of the arm might be elicited by noxious stimulation of the lower cervical dermatomes and from all thoracic sensory dermatomes 6 hours after an ictus. These reflex movements, elicitable in about 30% of cerebral death suspects at some time, presumably are evidence of receding spinal shock. Fine muscle twitchings, commonly referred to as muscle artifact, observed in the electroencephalogram were seen in more than half of the cases when no discernible bioelectric activity was present. This would tend to refute the hypothesis suggested by some electroencephalographers that these are dependent upon bulbar reflex activity.

Discussion

Theoretically, since cerebral death is the permanent cessation of brain function, the basic criteria should assess the activity of the cerebral hemispheres and the brainstem. Even a cursory survey of the data just reviewed confirms the early impression that coma and apnea are the two most sensitive indicators of cerebral death. In the absence of one or both of these findings, there may be irreparable and irreversible brain damage, but not a dead brain. The presence of these two clinical manifestations does not unequivocally indicate cerebral death, for there may be other evidence of activity in the brain. Yet, the two constitute a sensitive combination of clinical signs of cerebral death; for this reason, their absence is useful to screen brain death suspects.

The duration of coma and apnea sufficient to arouse suspicion of cerebral death may be estimated by analysis of the finding in 844 patients who were being considered as possible candidates for cerebral death. It was the impression of the attending physician that all of these patients at one time had had coma and apnea, although subsequent determinations did not

Table III-11.   The Course After Initial Coma and Apnea.

	Number of living patients at designated time		
Initial	After 15 minutes	After 1 hour	After 24 hours
844	503*	470**	392***

*341 patients initially considered comatose and apneic, no longer met these criteria.

**29 patients considered comatose and apneic after 15 minutes' observation regained consciousness or respiration within 1 hour; 4 patients died.

***48 patients considered comatose and apneic after 15 minutes' observation regained consciousness or respiration within 24 hours; 63 patients died.

Table III–12.   Time from Insult to Cerebral Unresponsivity and Apnea.

Elapsed Time	Cerebral Unresponsivity	Apnea
1.9 hrs.	333 cases	219
2–3.9	22	34
4–7.9	13	44
8–15.9	10	33
16–31.9	23 ⎫	
32 hrs. to 2 days	11 ⎬	59
>2 days	58	83
Unknown	33	31
Total	503	503

Table III–13.   Clinical Criteria in Brain Death (Modified from Allen et al.[9]).

Criteria	Correlation	Rapid Return in Survivors
Recommended		
Coma	+ + + +	+
Apnea	+ + + +	+
Absence of light reflex	+ + +	+
Absence of vestibular reflex*	+ + +	
Absence of oculocepahlic reflex	+ + +	
Absence of corneal reflex	+ + +	+
Desirable		
Spontaneous movements	+ +	+

*Not examined by some clinicians

necessarily confirm this opinion. Table III-11 gives the number of patients who would have qualified if the required time of coma and apnea for a cerebral death suspect had been 15 minutes, one hour and 24 hours. It is seen that if the required period is 15 minutes, a considerable number of patients who had only momentary apnea or coma are eliminated, leaving the more severe cases. Requiring one hour of coma and apnea reduces the population approximately 4% more, and 24 hours drops the number in the population by another 10%. It would therefore seem that a period of coma and apnea for 15 minutes eliminates most of the persons with transitory loss of cerebral function; increasing the time further does not appreciably improve the accuracy of the screening, but it does reduce the population by those dying within the waiting period.

The unresponsiveness and apnea often occur concomitantly shortly after the cerebral insult, but when they are dissociated, impaired consciousness tends to precede respiratory arrest (Table III-12). Rarely does the reverse occur, although it may do so when the principal insult is to the brainstem, leaving the cerebral cortex relatively uninjured. This state occurred in 2 of 53 cerebral death cases reported by Gaches et al. (141); isolated cases have also appeared in medical literature. (60)

Allen et al. (9), on the basis of their mathematical analyses, identified the clinical criteria of greatest value in the determination of cerebral death (Table III-13). Coma and apnea were inherent in the definition. The states of the light, vestibular, oculocephalic and corneal reflexes were considered to be of greatest value. The absence of these reflexes had a high discriminative power with cerebral death. Spontaneous movement, which correlated particularly highly 24 hours after the ictus, was considered slightly less valuable. The researchers considered that electrocerebral silence should be required for the diagnosis of brain death.

Chapter IV

Cerebral Circulation in Cerebral Death

Introduction

It has long been known that the brain has limited tolerance to interruption of its blood supply. In fact, total deprivation for less than a minute renders it functionless. The susceptibility of the brain to circulatory arrest is determined by its temperature, metabolic requirements, and other factors. Under normal internal and external environmental conditions, complete interruption of the cerebral circulation for a period of 5 minutes irreparably damages the brain. In experimental animals and man, a fall in cerebral blood flow (CBF) of even 50% depletes the high energy phosphates, and the brain cannibalizes itself.

Wertheimer et al. (510), noting that *coma dépassé* was accompanied by an arrest of cerebral circulation, concluded that cerebral death represented total cerebral infarction.

Cerebral Blood Flow

The cerebral blood flow depends upon the perfusion pressure, the viscosity of the blood and the vascular resistance.

Cerebral Perfusion Pressure. Cerebral perfusion pressure is defined as the difference between the mean systemic arterial blood pressure and the cerebral venous pressure. Thus, other factors remaining equal, cerebral perfusion pressure decreases with either a fall of the mean systemic arterial blood pressure (SAP) or a rise in intracranial pressure (ICP). The *critical cerebral perfusion pressure* may be defined as the lowest perfusion pressure capable of maintaining sufficient cerebral blood flow to meet the minimal metabolic requirements of the brain and to wash out products of degradation.

As early as 1902, Cushing (113) observed through a glass window in the calvarium of a monkey the blanching of vessels on the surface of the brain as an expanding intradural balloon increased the intracranial pressure. Recently, French investigators (163) have confirmed this finding with both contrast and isotope angiography. Brierley et al., (67) reported that irreversible brain damage was produced in monkeys when the perfusion pressure was lowered to 25 mm Hg if cerebral vascular autoregulatory mechanisms were abolished. Ingvar et al. (205) increased the intracranial pressure in a stepwise fashion until autoregulation was overcome and cerebral blood flow was reduced. This occurred at levels of intracranial pressure over 100 mm Hg, which corresponded to perfusion pressures below 40 mm Hg.

In a series of 10 cases of cerebral death, Balslev-Jorgensen et al. (30) found that the mean intracranial pressure (ICP) rose at some time above the mean systolic pressure (SAP). As the ICP/SAP ratio approached unity, Jorgensen (225) observed that the clinical state of the patient suddenly deteriorated, intracranial pulsations decreased in amplitude and ceased, and all clinical and electroencephalographic signs of brain function disappeared. In four cases of brain death, Riishede and Jacobsen (396) found that the ICP/SAP ratio was close to unity. However, in 5 other cases the perfusion pressure was 10–130 mm Hg, so that the arrest of cerebral circulation was not solely due to the low perfusion pressure. DeRougemont et al. (117) made simultaneous readings of the ICP and SAP in 38 persons suspected of cerebral death. The ICP/SAP ratio was 0.8–0.9 in 8 cases, 0.9–1.1 in 28, and 0.7 and 1.17 in the other 2 cases. In the routine neurosurgical case, even with high intracranial pressure from a tumor, the ratio rarely exceeds 0.5.

Viscosity of the Blood. Little attention has been given to the physical state of the blood in patients with cerebral death. Perhaps insufficient attention has been paid to coagulopathy, for Kjeldsberg (248) states that disseminated intravascular thrombosis is a common finding, although, except in cases of direct injury to the arterial wall, clotting in the larger vessels is rarely seen.

Vascular Resistance.   The intravascular resistance to blood flow is difficult to determine since it is a function of a number of variables: caliber of vessel, the viscosity of the blood, the flow rate and, probably, other factors. The usual calculation based upon pressure drop, blood viscosity and flow rate gives only an approximation of the vascular resistance, even if the intracranial pressure is kept constant. Obviously, the situation becomes even more complex in cerebral death, which is characterized by endothelial cell swelling that not only changes the caliber of vessels but modifies the viscosity of the circulating fluid. It is generally assumed that local regulatory vasomotor functions maintain a fairly constant blood flow in spite of increased resistance until regional compensatory mechanisms are broken, when purely physical factors operate to regulate blood flow. At this time, resistance to intracranial flow may become greatly increased by the anoxic cellular changes occurring as the result of impaired or absent blood flow.

Determination of Cerebral Blood Flow in Cerebral Death

In European countries where the absence of cerebral blood flow is equated with brain death, numerous techniques have been proposed for the demonstration of cerebral perfusion.

The ideal method for the measurement of cerebral blood flow should have the following characteristics:

1. Be noninvasive and nonoffensive to the laity
2. Have clearcut and easily interpreted end points
3. Be clinically applicable in special care units
4. Require no special skills that cannot be acquired by hospital personnel
5. Measure both supra- and infratentorial blood flow
6. Be independent of the greatly increased flow and distended collateral channels of the external carotid system found in cases of cerebral death.

Although few methods meet these requirements, a number of techniques for directly or indirectly assessing cerebral blood flow approach these ideals.

Direct Methods of Cerebral Blood Flow Determination

Quantitative Measurements of Cerebral Blood Flow.   The standard methods for quantitative determinations of cerebral blood flow (CBF) require the measurements of non-diffusable substances in arterial blood and venous blood from the jugular bulb. The latter blood is derived mainly from the cerebral hemispheres, so that the determinations relate to blood circulation of the supratentorial structures and not that of the brain stem or cerebellum. This anatomical arrangement of the cerebral circulation is disturbed in cases of cerebral death. In the first place, when the intracranial circulation is arrested, the augmented extracranial circulation (under greatly increased pressure) will probably increase the size of collateral channels and create new pathways for venous return. Hence, the jugular bulb will receive from its extracranial tributaries—meningeal, pharyngeal and emissary veins—a large volume of blood from the head, thus changing it from predominantly an intracranial to an extracranial sink of blood. Kety (241) states that only 2.7% of the blood in the superior jugular bulb is derived from extracerebral sources under normal circumstances. However, when the intracranial circulation is blocked and a pint and a half of blood each minute must be shunted into external channels, the percentage may be much higher—in fact, according to Brock et al.(70), three or four times that amount. In line with this statement, Riishede and Ethelberg (395) noted that in their first case there was dense filling of the diploic veins. The new blood channels and their altered physiology introduce problems in interpreting the results of determinations of cerebral blood flow that are dependent upon measurements of intracranial blood in the jugular bulb. In addition, the circulation of the jugular system is slowed because of the lack of visa tergo, and techniques requiring a mechanical wash-off, such as the mass spectrometer, may be rendered inoperative. Thus, the majority of the standard methods requiring the jugular bulb as a source of data are likely to be adversely influenced.

A second consideration, when intracarotid injections or flows are essential to the examination, is the possibility of extracerebral filling, either through the external carotid or ophthalmic arteries. In patients with no angiographically measurable intracerebral flow, Hadjidimos et al. (167) found CBF values of 7–15 ml/100 gm/min when ^{133}Xe was injected into the carotid artery; but when the arteries were exposed in the neck and the external carotid ligated, an injection into the internal carotid artery gave flow values too low to measure. The ophthalmic artery is another source of extracranial contamination. This is obvious (1) from its demonstration after intracarotid injections that show no intracranial circulation, (2) from the appearance of a bluish discoloration of the supraorbital region when Evans blue is injected in the carotid artery (used by some European neurologists as proof of the placement of a needle), and (3) by the fact that when using intracarotid isotopes, the highest counts and fastest clearances are found above the orbit.

These extracranial channels, which tend to vitiate many of the techniques for qualitative or quantitative measurements of CBF, are probably responsible for the range of CBF values obtained in brain death cases that angiographically show no intracranial filling.

In view of these anatomical variations, low CBF rates in cases suspected of cerebral death may not indicate intracranial circulation. It is true that slow passage of contrast media is occasionally seen in cases of brain death, and perhaps some of the above cases of low flow rates may fall in that category, but the suspicion is strong that many are the result of collateral circulation.

Angiography. While precise and exquisite techniques have been developed for the quantitative determination of cerebral blood flow (373) they involve expensive and complicated equipment, and require considerable technical skill for placement of needles or cannulas in vessels, as well as expertise in the calculations of the amount of intracranial circulating blood. For these reasons, they are not available except in university or research centers. Accordingly, attention will be given only to those techniques that can be used in the general hospital with ordinary equipment and relatively untrained personnel.

Many clinicians believe that serial cerebral angiography is the decisive method of diagnosing cerebral death. Carotid angiography alone, commonly used in the past, does not visualize the circulation of the brainstem and posterior fossa structures, and accordingly is inadequate for the proof of cerebral death. The demonstration of both the carotid and vertebrobasilar systems may be achieved by several methods: (1) selective catheterization of all four arteries by femoral or axillary artery puncture; (2) direct puncture of the carotid and the vertebral arteries; and (3) cerebral panarteriography by injection of contrast media into the ascending aorta or by retrograde brachial injection.

With the instrumentation now available and the technical skills that have been developed, these procedures are relatively safe and simple. Femoral catheterization is commonly used in patients with cerebral death because the field in which the arterial puncture is carried out is well away from the head, where resuscitative procedures are in progress. Moreover, puncture and intubation of the femoral artery are relatively simple, and with X-ray control selective catheterization of the neck vessels can be accomplished without difficulty. The dye is usually injected under 2 or 3 atmospheres pressure and, because of the slowed circulation, serial films are taken over a somewhat longer period of time than when cerebral angiography is done under normal conditions.

Riishede and Jacobsen (396) advocate the Seldinger angiographic technique with a catheter passed through the femoral artery into the ascending aorta into which dye is injected under pressure. In 31 comatose and apneic patients (13 severe head injuries, 10 intracranial tumors and 8 vascular lesions), angiograms showed normal opacification of the aorta and its branches. The internal carotid and vertebral arteries filled very slowly and faintly; usually the dye tapered to a pointed end at varying distances from the base of the skull. In 30 cases, no dye entered the cranial cavity. In one case there was faint bilateral filling of the first portion of the anterior and middle cerebral arteries, seen 11 seconds after injection and 4 seconds after the dye had disappeared from the external carotid circulation. Greitz et al. (161) used aortocranioangiography in 42 patients, with or without additional selective unilateral injections. In all but one case they found contrast media arrested at the bifurcation of the carotid artery in the neck, at the siphon, or at the trunk of the middle cerebral artery. The advantages of injection into the aorta, Greitz et al.(161) claim, are its simplicity and the opacification of the external carotid circulation which serves as a control. Bradac and Simon (63) also believe that arch aortography is the method of choice. However, Busse and Vogelsang, (82) although considering it ideal for adults, question its use in children.

In cerebral death, the angiographic findings in the internal carotid artery may be of several types (161). Rarely there may be a tapering of the dye column in the cervical portion of the internal carotid artery, but more commonly a fairly abrupt block is seen at the cranial base or in the carotid siphon near the anterior or posterior clinoid process with or without visualization of the ophthalmic artery. In a few cases, there may be a delayed filling of the intracranial portion of the internal carotid artery with a slight density in the first part of the middle cerebral artery and rarely opacification of the anterior cerebral artery. The dye column usually arrests symmetrically in the carotid arteries, but occasionally it extends more distally on one side. In all cases, there is excellent and often premature visualization of the external carotid vessels. No intracranial venous phase, however, is ever observed (Figure IV-1).

The dye column in the vertebral artery is rarely blocked in the transversarial canal but usually is interrupted at the atlantooccipital junction, and less often intracranially. Occasionally a narrow streak of dye is seen in the basilar artery lying against the clivus, and the vertebral artery on the side opposite the injection may be visualized by retrograde filling. If there is not a complete block, the posterior cerebral and superior and inferior cerebellar arteries may be seen. The posterior communicating artery occasionally is opacified as far as the ipsilateral internal carotid artery. However, the circulation of the vertebrobasilar system is slow and there is no visualization of the venous channels.

An outstanding phenomenon is the marked contrast between the striking filling of the external carotid system and the delayed and poor influx into

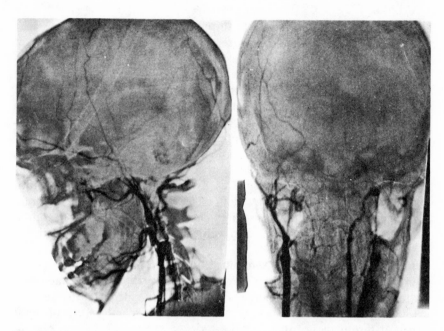

Fig. IV–1. Lateral and anteroposterior angiograms of a man with clinical manifestations of cerebral death as the result of salicylate intoxication. The aortic arch injection demonstrates the external carotid circulation but no intracranial flow from either the internal carotid or vertebral arteries (JJH).

the internal carotid artery. This difference between extra- and intracranial circulation is present but less prominent in the vertebrobasilar system. If intracerebral vascular filling occurs, the dye opacifies the vessels for a considerable time, lasting up to 30 minutes. The flow in the carotid and basilar systems may cease concurrently, but frequently the vertebrobasilar circulation persists for some hours after the carotid flow has stopped.

There is some evidence to suggest that as the pathophysiological processes associated with cerebral death progress, and intracranial pressure rises, there is less and less visualization of the intracranial portions of the vascular system, and eventually a block at the base of the skull. For this reason, Bücheler et al. (77) suggest that angiography should not be carried out soon after a clinical diagnosis of cerebral death even if the EEG is isoelectric, but should be deferred until the systemic circulation and the body temperature begin to fall and the A-V oxygen difference decreases.

Return of Cerebral Blood Flow.   Riishede and Ethelberg, (395) who first demonstrated this "nonfilling phenomenon" in five patients with supratentorial mass lesions producing increased intracranial pressure, emphasized that the stasis was not due to thrombosis of the cerebral vessels and, accordingly, in some cases the process might be reversible. A number of authors have reported such instances. In the cases reported by Riishede et al. (396) and Pribram, (384) removal of fluid by ventricular puncture so lessened the ICP that the cerebral vessels filled upon angiography and the patients recovered. Mitchell et al. (324) and Horwitz and Dunsmore (192) cite similar cases. Clar et al. (97) reported that after an intravenous infusion of sorbitol a previously nonfilling cerebral circulation could be demonstrated. In this case and those reported by Agnoli et al. (4) there must have been some intracranial flow to allow the hypertonic solutions to act upon the cerebral hemispheres. However, in practice, such return of cerebral circulation is usually ineffective in restoring an ischemic brain to a functional state. Still, the isolated demonstration of arrest of cerebral circulation cannot be considered unequivocal evidence of brain death.

Errors in Interpretation of Nonfilling of Intracranial Vessels.   Errors in interpretation may result from slow or diffuse circulation, the faulty injection of the dye (subintimally instead of intraluminally), a marked fall in blood pressure, often associated with brachycardia and, rarely, bilateral spasm or thrombosis of the carotid arteries.

Vlahovitch (485) emphasized that a negative finding is not conclusive and that positive evidence of absent CBF should be demonstrated. To this end, he injects the intracarotid dye under pressure (3.5 kg, or twice that attained by hand) so as to ensure opacification of the cerebral vessels. He and his collaborators (488) report that at a pressure of 2.5 to 3.5 kg it is possible to fill carotid and vertebral arteries with dye that stagnates in these vessels for 4 to 20 minutes, gradually passing to extracranial arteries and in 25% of cases to the venous sinuses. They consider retention of the dye in the cerebral vessels for 2 or more minutes to be proof of arrested circulation. By cineradiography of the cerebral circulation, Decker and Kunkel (115) demonstrated that total cessation of circulation was less common than reduced cerebral blood flow in the early phases of cerebral death.

Comment.   The use of contrast angiography to assist in making a diagnosis of brain death has only recently gained popularity in the United States. The fear of possible complications is not well founded. Feild et al. (131) found a mortality rate of 0.34% per arteriogram performed among 2000 consecutive patients; these were primarily percutaneous carotid angiograms. They found a complication rate of 0.21% among 1000 consecutive cases undergoing retrograde brachial arteriograms (132). The fear of complications arises primarily because the risk of arteriography has not been established in patients who have both a severe neurological debility and also a greatly slowed cerebral circulation (361), for the toxic effects of contrast materials may be substantially greater when they are in contact with cerebral vessels for a prolonged period of time.

Isotope Angiography.   Isotope angiography, introduced by Maynard et al. (311) in 1969, provides a noninvasive means of grossly evaluating cerebral circulation. A number of variations of this general technique have been used. Both the rectilinear scan and imaging camera are capable of showing isotope activity in blood vessels and sinuses within the skull; an empty scan indicates a lack of cerebral blood flow. The obvious advantage of these techniques is the simplicity and atraumatic nature of the examination. Unfortunately, both external and internal carotid circulations are demonstrated and so a quantitative measurement of CBF is difficult. The inability to differentiate internal from external carotid circulation is a serious disadvantage, for although under normal circumstances the external circulation may amount to only 5–9 ml/100 gm/min, according to Brock et al. (70) if the internal flow is dammed the collateral external circulation may be greatly increased.

Intravenous Techniques.   The technique used by Maynard and his associates (311) involves the intravenous injection of 15 millicuries of sodium pertechnetate (99m Tc) as a bolus into an antecubital vein. After a five-second delay, polaroid films are exposed every 3 seconds for 24 seconds with an Anger camera positioned over the forehead. Using this technique. Goodman et al. (156) report that in over 500 consecutive isotope angiograms the major cerebral arteries and dural sinuses filled in all but 3 cases, which had clinical evidence of brain death. In a later publication, they refer to 18 empty cranial cavities in 4,000 radionuclide angiograms (323). The authors admit that the method gives only a crude measure of the cerebral circulation and lacks both the high resolution of contrast angiography and the ability to produce quantitative estimates of CBF, but they consider it a sensitive and definitive means of determining an absent cerebral blood flow. Ouaknine et al. (361) have emphasized the markedly slowed circulation that may be demonstrated with this technique, the isotope remaining in the cerebral vessels for 15 minutes in some cases. Using an intravenous radionuclide technique with a conventional linear scanner, they found that the uptake of the isotope was confined to the territory of the external carotid artery—scalp, temporalis muscle and neck musculature. This localization of the isotope and the absence of activity over the superior longitudinal and lateral sinuses they consider to be the hallmarks of an absent cerebral blood flow (Figure IV–2).

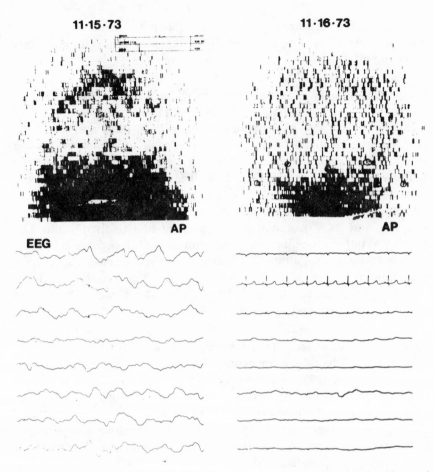

Fig. IV–2. Isotopic scans of a patient with meningoencephalitis and clinical evidence of cerebral death.
A   Normal intracranial flow pattern and biological activity in the EEG flow pattern.
B   Empty scan on the following day and ECS (Courtesy of Dr. E. B. Schlesinger).

Bolus Technique.   The bolus technique is a nonquantitative, time/activity curve of the initial head passage of an intravenously injected radioisotope bolus. A rapid intravenous injection of 2 mCi of 99 mTc O_4 in 2 cc of saline is delivered in the antecubital vein. A single cephalic probe with a collimator so designed as to limit the field of view to the cerebral structures above the floor of the skull is placed in contact with the midline of the forehead. Thus, most or all of the posterior fossa is outside the field. A second probe is placed over a pulsating femoral artery, located by palpation, to serve as a control. Without clear evidence of a compact bolus in the femoral artery, no reliance can be placed on absence of the head bolus (Figure IV–3).

Korein et al. (255) report on 142 bolus studies on 80 suspect brain death patients. Considering only those cases in which a satisfactory control curve was obtained, two different time/activity curves of the head area were obtained.

One type of tracing, a "bolus curve", shows a relatively sharp rise and fall of recorded radioactivity in both cephalic and femoral records, and presumably represents the injected bolus passing through the cerebral and systemic circulations; these are not distinguishable from tracings obtained in noncomatose patients. They indicate sufficient cerebral blood flow for maintenance of a viable but not necessarily a normal cerebrum. In sharp contrast, a second type of head tracing displays a gradual low magnitude linear increase in radioisotopic activity and a normal femoral bolus curve. No distinct peak is observed in the cephalic trace during the minute fol-

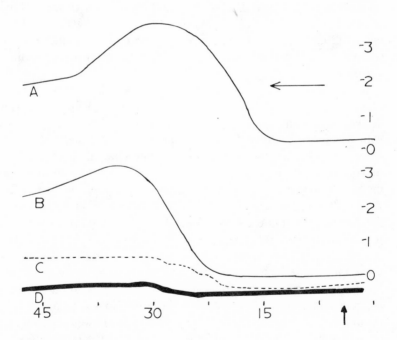

Fig. IV–3. Bolus curves to show:

A   Normal cephalic curve.
B   Normal curve from femoral artery.
C   Interrupted line—intermediate cephalic curve probably representing no CBF.
D   Heavy line—flat cephalic tracing with no curve representing absence of CBF.
The figures at the right are counts ($\times 10^5$) per minute. At the base, the arrow represents the time of injection; the markers represent the time in seconds. (redrawn from originals)

lowing the injection. This type of head time/activity tracing is considered to indicate a grossly deficient cerebral circulation. The delayed low level and gradual buildup in activity probably represent radionuclide activity in the extracerebral circulation. Of the 80 deeply comatose and apneic patients fulfilling the basic criteria for suspicion of cerebral death, 27 had evidence on all their radioisotopic flow examinations of the presence of a cephalic bolus. All but three of these patients had electrical activity in their EEGs, the exceptions being patients in whom repeated EEGs were technically unsatisfactory. Five of the 27 patients with drug-induced coma survived and became neurologically normal.

Quantitative determinations of CBF were made in some cases; the lowest CBF associated with a bolus-type curve was 24% of normal flow. Since in coma vigil the CBF is reduced to 25%, one might assume that this is the minimal CBF that could sustain cerebral metabolism—and that at this level a bolus curve would be present.

In 37 patients, the cerebral bolus effect was absent, and of these 31 patients had isoelectric EEGs prior and subsequent to the radioisotopic tests. All 37 patients died; 23 had spontaneous, irreversible cardiac arrest, and in 12 cases resuscitation procedures were discontinued; in 2 others it was not clear whether resuscitation was discontinued or cardiac arrest occurred.

In 4 additional patients with adequately controlled isotopic flow studies, an intermediate response with a slow rise in the cephalic tracing was qualitatively different from the type I and II traces. However, all 4 patients with this type of curve had an isoelectric EEG and died. In one patient, a four-vessel angiogram demonstrated no intracranial flow from the carotid or vertebral arteries. For these reasons, the authors consider the intermediate response as equivalent to a no-bolus curve.

The other 12 patients were considered to have unsatisfactory flow studies, due to inadequate femoral controls, inadvertent injection of radioisotopes into the femoral artery or too slow injection of the radioisotope into the intravenous line. In some cases, both femoral arteries were inaccessible since they were being used for intravenous fluids or were covered by bandages or casts. Other reasons for a technically unsatisfactory bolus study included shock and errors in calibration. In 4 patients with no bolus or intermediate traces, four-vessel angiography showed virtually no intracranial filling, except for one case with markedly delayed filling of the posterior circulation.

The authors consider this examination to be a simple, innocuous bedside test for cerebral circulation. Any error, they believe, would always be on the side of misdiagnosing a dead cerebrum as alive. This technique does not detect flow through the posterior fossa structures, but the authors believe this is not disadvantageous, for they consider that cerebral death implies only destruction of the cerebral hemispheres.

Intra-Arterial Techniques.   Several investigators have used tracer clearance techniques to measure regional cerebral blood flow (rCBF) in patients with brain death. In two cases, Bes et al. (47) utilized a percutaneous intracarotid injection of ^{133}Xe, and external counting to obtain average blood flows of 7 and 11 ml/100g/min respectively. However, much or all of this flow may be due to regurgitation from the internal to the external carotid artery, for Brock et al. (70) have shown that even when the external carotid artery is digitally compressed during the injection some tracer regurgitates. When an injection of isotope was made directly into a surgically exposed internal carotid artery, only a small amount of tracer entered the brain, much less reached the cerebral cortex, and virtually none of it was cleared during more than thirty minutes of external monitoring. A number of French investigators have studied the transit curves after carotid injection of isotopes. Baldy-Moulinier and Frérebeau, (29) who percutaneously injected ^{133}Xe into the internal carotid arteries of 9 patients in profound coma, found either a plateau or an initial peak followed by a plateau, which they considered to represent failure of clearance and a sign of circulatory arrest. Using an intracarotid injection of ^{133}Xe, and extracranial detectors, Deraux (116) reported curves of three types:

1. A flat trace indicating the failure of xenon to reach the cranial cavity

2. A plateau indicating some intracranial penetration but no clearance

3. Rarely, an initial spike presumably due to passage of the isotope through the basal vessels of the brain.

Lazorthe (276) studied 20 cases using this method and concluded that a flat trace indicated an arrest of cerebral circulation and cerebral death.

Intracerebral Techniques.   To eliminate the possibility of regurgitation to the external carotid circulation, Lazorthe and Bes (277) injected ^{133}Xe into the cerebral parenchyma and followed the clearance. They considered a plateau to indicate a lack of cerebral circulation and two such curves at ten-minute intervals a dead brain.

Zwetnow (527) injected krypton 85 intracerebrally through a previously placed burr hole in 40 cases and was able to demonstrate by external detectors that there was no clearance of the isotope in brains that had arrested circulation. Steinwall (450), using an isotope (^{75}Se) that was selectively taken up by the brain, thus avoiding contamination of the extracerebral tissues, studied the clearance of the isotope to determine the presence or absence of cerebral circulation.

Inhalation Techniques.   Hoyer and Wawersik (198) using the nitrous oxide clearance method of Kety and Schmidt in four patients with clinical evidence of brain death, found a mean CBF of 15.2 ml/100 g/min. Shalit et al. (425), with the same technique, found a mean CBF of 9.1 ml/100 g/min in three patients with brain death. They pointed out, however, that the uptake of nitrous oxide was not complete because of slow flow, and consequently the CBF values were not accurate. Techniques requiring jugular blood are subject to misinterpretation, for the venous samples, when there is essentially no intracranial flow, would not be expected to be representative of the cerebral blood. Nor is the flow demonstrated by a hydrogen electrode necessarily representative of blood flow in the entire cerebrum, since this technique only samples the local oxygen tension (226).

Computerized tomography.   With the greatly increased use of computerized tomography in all patients with suspected intracranial lesions, a new technique for the demonstration of cerebral blood flow has become available in all the larger hospitals. Although the computerized scan does not show normal blood vessels, the enhanced scan, which is almost routinely used, does visualize the major intracranial vessels. Thus, the inability to see the intracranial portion of the internal carotid artery in such scans is evidence of the lack of intracranial circulation.

Indirect Methods of Determining Cerebral Blood Flow

Rheoencephalography.   Studies by Kramer and Tuyman (263) with intracerebral electrodes have indicated that the rheoencephalogram becomes flat at the same time as the EEG when the intracranial pressure approximates the arterial tension; when the pressure is lowered, the rheoencephalogram tends to return to normal before the EEG. Lanner and Argyrepoulos (273) correlated impedance studies with other methods of studying brain activity, and concluded that rheoencephalography added a refinement to the diagnosis of cerebral death. However, surface recordings do not always correspond to depth impedance studies, so that complete reliance cannot be placed on clinical rheoencephalograms for the diagnosis of cerebral death.

Echoencephalography.   The presence or absence of cerebral circulation may be determined by the simple and noninvasive echoencephalographic demonstration of an intracranial vascular pulsation. Leksell (281) in his early description of echoencephalography described a midline pulsatile echo that was synchronous with the heart beat. The echo pulsation seen on the cathode ray screen becomes a quasi-sinusoidal wave when recorded on a time scale by an inkwriter. Although the midline pulsating echoes are the most prominent and most commonly studied in echoencephalography, pulsating echoes may be demonstrated throughout the brain substance. These zonal pulsations in the brain are depicted by gating any desired portion of the reflected echo. LePetit et al. (282) have recorded the signals at 1 cm intervals throughout the hemisphere. Such hemispheral pulsations are almost entirely due to carotid shock waves, whereas the midline pulsations are in part derived from basilar pulsations. Accordingly, the hemispheral pulsations may be absent while the midline pulsations persist. For this reason some investigators (282) have used the absence of the hemispheral pulsations as evidence of cerebral death, and others (470) have recorded midline pulsations in the belief that they are more sensitive indicators of cerebral circulation. The proof that these pulsations are related to cerebral blood flow stems from both clinical and experimental studies. LePetit et al. (282), using cinematographic methods, have shown that the intracranial pulsatile echo is not seen when cerebral blood flow cannot be demonstrated by angiography. Marusasa (305), who studied the relationships of the brain pulsations to clinical and angiograhic findings in animals and man, found that the flat echo pulsation curve coincided with nonfilling of the cerebral vessels in angiograms. Other clinical studies have confirmed the absence of brain pulsations when cerebral circulation is obstructed.

Arnold et al. (24) noted that midline echo pulsations may still be detected after cerebral circulation can no longer be demonstrated angiographically. This effect was probably due to pulsations in the stems of the carotid and basilar arteries, even though blood did not pass through them. Moreover, Arnold et al. (24) reported that in a comatose patient the echoes from the lateral ventricles pulsated but those from the midline did not. An examination of the tracings showed that the midline echoes were pathological and probably represented reflections from hemorrhagic or lacerated tissue rather than the third ventricular walls. LePetit et al. (283), who consider that an absence of hemispheral pulsatile echoes is evidence of arrest of carotid circulation and implies irreversible loss of cerebral function, have evaluated over 100 patients in stage IV coma (apneic, unresponsive and without cephalic reflexes) with a flat EEG. They were unable to find any hemispheric pulsations even with multidirectional recordings. In no case was there a return of pulsations once they disappeared. In those cases in which carotid angiography was carried out, the films showed exo- or endocranial stasis of the dye in the internal carotid arteries. In 7 cases of toxic coma with similar clinical findings, there were persistent pulsatile echoes in the cerebral hemispheres. The authors admit that vertebrobasilar echoes may be detected for some time after the cessation of hemispheral pulsatile echoes. They conclude that the presence of three criteria—stage IV coma, a flat EEG tracing and immobile hemispheral echoes—is sufficient to prove the death of the brain (283).

Uematsu et al. (470) used an ultrasonic reflectoscope with a 2.0 MHz piezoelectric transducer and a gating system for display of the echo signal in one channel of an electroencephalograph. In order to record the signal for more careful analysis, they separated and isolated the appropriate echo from the other signals by using an electronic switch controlled by a pulse generator to give any desired width at any time. The gated midline echo was converted to a sequence of pulses, each of which was proportional in amplitude to the appropriate echo pulse, but spanned half of the 2.5 millisecond pulse-to-pulse interval. The resulting signal could be recorded on any strip chart recorder, oscillograph or EEG pen writer. As many such gates as desired could be constructed to allow the simultaneous recording of the pulsatile component of two or more echoes. To ensure stability o. the transducer, a head band and holder were devised so that the ultrasonic transducer could be adjusted manually and maintained in an appropriate position (Figure IV-4).

Patients with normal cerebral blood flow invariably had a pulsation of the midline echo. Uematsu et al. reported on 45 comatose cases using this technique. A normal pulsatile midline echo was present in 3 obtunded and 15 comatose patients and in 2 of 27 cases suspected of cerebral death. In the remaining 25 cases of cerebral death the midline echoes did not pulsate. There was an absence of echo pulsation in all 4 patients suspected of brain death in whom angiograms showed non-filling of the intracranial blood vessels.

The dissociated findings of an isoelectric encephalogram and a pulsating echo may be the result of an ischemic brain still being irrigated, of pulsations arising from the stump of an occluded carotid or basilar artery, or of a fall in perfusion pressure sufficient to abolish the electroencephalogram but still adequate to produce pulsations detectable by echography. It is well known that the biological activity of the EEG may disappear as the blood pressure falls to subshock levels, then reappear when vasopressors elevate the BP to near normal levels. In the cases of dissociated findings in Uematsu et al.'s series, the arterial pressure was fluctuating from imperceptible to shock levels. This severe hypotension apparently was inadequate to sustain neuronal activity, but sufficient to produce shock waves capable of distorting the walls of the third ventricle.

Uniform changes in the consistency of cerebral tissues, severe anemia, dehydration, inflammatory process or edema may not significantly affect the echo, but liquefaction of the brain during deanimation may abolish

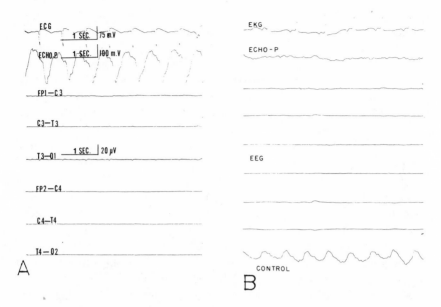

Fig. IV–4. Echoencephalogram and electroencephalogram traces to show:

A Channel
1. electrocardiogram
2. normal echoencephalogram
3–8. absence of biological activity

B Channel
1. electrocardiogram
2. absence of the midline echo
3–8. absence of biological activity
9. A record of the echoencephalogram of a normal control using the same settings as in Channel 2. (JHH)

echoes. However, this finding is less common in cerebral death than the absence of the midline pulsation.

Ophthalmic Artery Blood Flow. Since the ophthalmic artery is given off just after the internal carotid enters the cranium, several investigators have attempted to use the state of the retinal circulation as an index of flow in the intracranial portions of the internal carotid arteries. Direct observation of the retinal flow is possible by ophthalmoscopy, (374) at least in the early stages of cerebral death. Later, the cornea may become milky and opaque as it dries out or is covered with ointments to prevent drying. However, at the initial examination, especially if the pupils are dilated and fixed, the fundi are readily inspected. The retinal vessels may have a slowed circulation with sludging of erythrocytes or complete cessation of circulation, in which event the clumped erythrocytes appear like strings of sausages in the vessels. Unfortunately, sludging is not very common in the retinae of patients with a dead brain. Of 98 cases examined in the Collaborative

Study, only 20 had sludging. As a corollary to clinical studies of retinal circulation, Vlahovitch and Boudet (486) examined the ophthalmic circulation by carotid angiography. In about half of 25 cases of deep coma, persistent opacification of the choroidal crescent and ophthalmic artery indicated circulatory arrest. Thus, although the ocular supply is derived in part, at least, from extracranial sources, it is often arrested in cerebral death.

Lobstein et al. (294) and Mantz et al. (303) have studied the arm-retinal circulation time using fluorescein injected by a catheter into the subclavian vein while the retinal vessels were being observed ophthalmoscopically. Because the circulation time was greatly increased from the normal of 8–14 seconds in two thirds of 33 cases of *coma dépassé*, they concluded that a circulation time greater than 30 seconds was a certain sign of *coma dépassé*. Derangements of ophthalmic artery flow may be shown by a Doppler directional flow meter in cases of brain death (339). Using ultrasonography, Despland and De Crousaz (119) believe that they can diagnose cerebral death on the basis of a complex of findings, namely, (1) a high systolic flow in the carotid arteries with replacement of the continuous diastolic flow by a reversal of flow in part of diastole, and (2) a lack of (in the case of cerebral lesions) or an intermittent (in posterior fossa lesions) orthodromic flow in the ophthalmic artery. Other methods which could be used for this purpose but have not been reported to date include ophthalmodynamometry and the use of thermistors or thermography to determine the presence or absence of blood flow in the supraorbital branches of the ophthalmic arteries. These techniques, although requiring special equipment and a certain expertise, are simple, harmless and, if positive, would give confirmatory evidence of the arrest of cerebral circulation.

Electroretinography.   In cases of cerebral death, Mantz et al. (303) found that the waves of the electroretinogram (ERG) are affected differentially by retinal ischemia; the "a" wave is resistent and the "b" wave quite susceptible to anoxia. However, the ERG has been found to give inconsistent results in cerebral death with false positives, negatives, or confusing partial correlations. Sims et al. (437), using computer techniques to produce a 3-dimensional display (compressed spectral analysis) of the ERG, found that a brain death patient can have an ERG indistinguishable from that of an alert individual. Hence ERG cannot be recommended as a method to demonstrate cerebral death.

It would seem that brain death is difficult to confirm by observations based upon the ophthalmic circulation. Perhaps this should be expected, for it is well known that in 3% of cases the external carotid artery is the main source of blood to the ophthalmic artery and that the facial artery provides collateral circulation to the ophthalmic artery, so that retinal ischemia might not occur until the systemic circulation failed. Hence definitive evidence of absence of cerebral circulation based upon ophthalmic findings would be present in only a small percentage of patients.

Chapter V

Biochemical Findings in Cerebral Death

Diagnosis of the Primary Condition

In the study of comatose persons, the clinical laboratory is valuable both in the diagnosis of the primary disorder and in the establishment of the death of the brain. Among the common disorders that produce clinical states resembling those of a dead brain are the intoxicating agents, mainly sedative drugs. The recognition of these reversible states depends upon the diagnostic acumen of the attending physician and the accuracy of the clinical laboratory (499).

Drug Intoxications. The suspicion of a drug ingestion is aroused by the environment about a comatose patient. The presence of a suicide note or an empty or partially full bottle of sedative medication is an obvious suggestion that a drug is responsible. Needle puncture wounds in the flexor surface of the forearm, especially the left, is another indication. However, any individual, particularly a young one, found in a comatose state should arouse the suspicion that drugs may be responsible. Yet, even under research conditions, physicians frequently fail to consider the possibility of drugs and to take blood for chemical analysis. In the Collaborative Study, although required by protocol, for many reasons—some related to therapeutic endeavors, some to inadequate local facilities, and many, probably, due to simple failure to collect blood—determinations of blood levels were obtained in just over half of the cases (313 of 503). Even in 61 cases with some historical or circumstantial evidence of drug abuse, such as a suicide note or an empty bottle of pills, no reports of the barbiturate levels were available in 17 patients (28%). In all, 62 patients, some admittedly with obvious lethal neurological conditions, were declared "cerebrally dead" without benefit of a drug survey. Although no patient with a history of drug intoxication was pronounced a cerebral death without a local barbiturate analysis, five patients with drug intoxications did die from cardiac arrest without having had blood assays. On the other hand, 26 of the 252 patients not clinically suspected to have ingested drugs were found to have levels of sedative drugs in the blood in the same range of magnitude as those of the 61 intoxicated patients.

Not only is there the risk that blood may not be submitted to the laboratory, but there is also the question of the accuracy of the determinations. In the Collaborative Study, levels of the sedative drugs in blood, plasma or serum were determined at a central laboratory. Phenobarbital was most frequently found; its highest concentration was 185 μm/ml. A few other sedatives were present in the blood of some patients. One patient had 200 μm/ml of meprobamate, a concentration compatible with deep central nervous depression. High concentrations of ethchlorvynol, glutethimide and alcohol were also found in a few patients. Comparison of the barbiturate levels reported by local and central laboratories of split samples of blood were made in 175 cases. In comparing the barbiturate determinations, the results were considered to agree if the center data differed by no more than $\pm$ 5 μg/ml from the control results. The findings are shown in the histogram (Figure V–1). If one laboratory reported that no drug was present in the blood, the other laboratory usually had similar findings (131 cases); in only two cases in which the central laboratory found no barbiturates did the local laboratories report significant levels (20 μg/ml), and in another two cases in which the hospitals reported no barbiturates the central laboratory found significant amounts.

Of the 44 patients having barbiturates in the blood assays at both local and central laboratories, 19 individuals had levels that differed more than 5 μg/ml. In nine of these cases, the results varied more than 15 μg/ml. That these discrepancies may have been due to differences in time at which the blood was drawn for analysis seems unlikely; the variations in time were about the same as in the cases with levels within 5 μg/ml. In four instances, the blood was taken at the same time, and differences from -16 to $+40$ μg/ml were found. In one case, the local determination was 20 μg/ml, and the central laboratory reported no barbiturates in blood taken 75 minutes later; in another case in which blood samples were taken within 5 hours, the difference was 39 μg/ml. In two cases, the time of blood withdrawal was not reported. In one case, the local analysis was made on blood obtained 24 hours before the sample for the central lab-

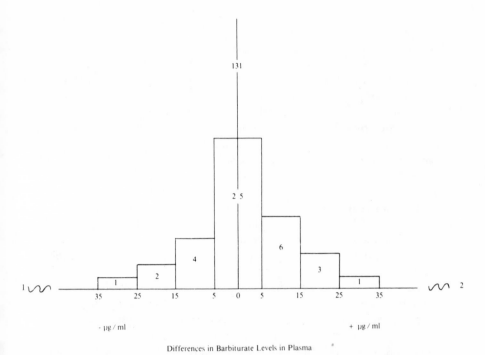

131

2 5

6

4

3

2

1

1

1

35   25   15   5   0   5   15   25   35

- µg / ml

+ µg / ml

Differences in Barbiturate Levels in Plasma

Fig. V–1. Histogram to show the differences in µg/ml between barbiturate levels as reported by local and central laboratories. The results of the central laboratory are the standard against which the local findings are compared. Only differences greater than 5.0 µg/ml are recorded. At zero on the abscissa are 131 cases reported by the two laboratories to have no barbiturates in the plasma; in the central histogram are 25 cases in which barbiturate levels are determined by the two laboratories differed by no more than 5.0 µg/ml. In the remaining cases, differences as plotted were reported. To the right of the zero ordinate, the histograms indicate the number of cases with higher values (to the extent indicated) reported by the local than the central laboratory. To the left of the zero ordinate are the cases with lower values reported by the local laboratory.

oratory was taken at autopsy 2 hours after death. The initial level was 45 ± 15 µg/ml, and the latter 13 µg/ml.

The differences in the results occurred at all blood levels of barbiturates as determined at the central laboratory.

Other problems unrelated to the accuracy of the level of drugs in the blood frequently complicate the making of a diagnosis. Although in the Collaborative Study more than half of the patients with drug(s) in the blood succumbed, few had blood levels in the lethal range. Even the drug levels in deeply comatose patients were rarely in the accepted toxic range— for phenobarbital, 53–170 µg/ml blood (459). In fact, the majority of the levels were no higher than those considered to be in the therapeutic range for epilepsy (Table V–1). Edwards et al. (127) have also noted a low barbiturate level (1.4μg/ml) in a comatose patient.

A number of possible factors may account for the poor correlation between the blood level and the clinical state. The time of drawing the blood after ingestion of phenobarbital, which has a half-life of approximately 72 hours, would seem to be an unlikely factor. Potentiation of the effect of the barbiturates by other drugs or conditions may play a role in the dissociation between blood level and pharmacological effect. Head injuries causing cerebral edema, or systemic conditions that modify the permeability of the blood brain barrier, may increase the tissue concentration of the drug. In view of the above uncertainties, to make a diagnosis of poisoning does not require the demonstration of toxic blood levels; the presence of even a small amount of a sedative agent should alert the physician to initiate treatment promptly for an intoxication.

In spite of the deficiencies and possible sources of error, it seems unlikely that many drug-intoxicated patients were missed in the Collaborative Study. Moreover, if drugs were present, cases in which the local barbiturate determinations were the same or higher than those at the central laboratory caused no serious error; only those cases with lower levels reported by the local laboratories might have been misinterpreted and mismanaged. There were nine cases in which this type of error may have occurred; in seven cases some barbiturate was recorded. However, since the possibility of serious consequences remained in this carefully supervised series, it must be admitted that routine drug analyses probably have even greater danger of error.

Twenty-six patients, unsuspected of drug intoxication but found by the central laboratory to have detectable amounts of sedative drugs, had other primary diagnoses. Although in some cases these drugs may have been administered for therapeutic reasons, the fact that such cases were encountered points out that the effects of a reversible pharmacological factor may be masked by the catastrophic manifestations of a severe structural lesion and go unrecognized unless the patient's blood is screened for de-

Table V–1.   Relationship of Barbiturate Levels to Outcome.

Level (μg/ml)	Survived	Died	Total
0–9	6	9	15
10–29	8	4	12
30–59	3	3	6
60+	5	—	5
Not done or Unknown	4	13	17
Other drug	4	2	6
Total	30	31	61

pressant drugs. Even then, since the techniques of analysis may not identify some toxic agents, the evaluation of the role of sedative drugs in comatose patients requires a high degree of suspicion and sound clinical judgment.

The Metabolic Diagnosis of Cerebral Death

As cerebral metabolism fails, oxygen is not consumed, CO_2 remains at a low level in the venous blood, and products of degradation accumulate. This constellation of chemical changes may be utilized in the determination of cerebral death.

Theoretically, a determination of cerebral metabolism ($CMRO_2$), the ultimate measure of function of the brain, appears to be the best available technique for the establishment of cerebral death. It is calculated from estimates of cerebral blood flow (CBF) and the arteriovenous difference of the O_2 content across the brain ($AVDO_2$). If the cerebral hemispheres have not extracted any, or have extracted only insignificant amounts of O_2 from the blood passing through them, they may be considered non-functional. The possibility that they are using their own proteins has little practical benefit, for the end product of amino-acid metabolism in the absence of oxidative processes is lactic acid, which results in an acidosis incompatible with metabolic enzyme activity. Although a low $CMRO_2$ indicates a nonfunctional cerebrum, proof that the brain is dead requires that the inactivity be present for a time that has been estimated experimentally from 5 minutes to as long as an hour.

The determination of $CMRO_2$ requires the placement of needles or catheters in the jugular bulb and in an artery, and the withdrawal of blood for analysis of O_2 and CO_2. This technique has two deficiencies: (1) the cerebral blood flow measurements cannot be obtained for the entire brain by current techniques; and (2) in the event of little or no cerebral blood flow, the blood obtained from the jugular bulb may not be representative of intracranial venous blood, but may be grossly contaminated by extra-cranial blood from the structures at the base of the skull (*see* chapter IV). For this reason, the $CMRO_2$ determinations in cerebral death suspects may be erroneously low.

Because the determination of the cerebral metabolic rate requires multiple vascular punctures and complicated equipment for the chemical assay of O_2 in arterial and venous blood, the technique is performed only in large medical centers and usually on a research basis. For this reason, relatively few reports of $CMRO_2$ determinations in cases of cerebral death have appeared.

The mass spectrometer is well suited to study cerebral blood flow and oxygen consumption since it is capable of performing both of these determinations repeatedly and simultaneously. Catheters are placed in a convenient artery, usually the femoral, and in the region of the jugular bulb. Arterial and venous determinations of argon gas allow calculation of cerebral blood flow using the Kety-Schmidt formula. Oxygen consumption is calculated from the values for cerebral blood flow and arteriovenous oxygen difference. The main problems in the use of this technique are decreasing sensitivity of the electrodes in time as a fibrin film forms on them and the possibility that jugular bulb blood does not accurately represent blood leaving the brain, but rather retrograde flow from the extracranial circulation. Pevsner et al.(373) found strikingly reduced levels of oxygen consumption in the two patients who had isoelectric EEGs, 0.6 and 0.0 mlO_2/100 gm/minute, respectively; they recommended $CMRO_2$ as a reliable method of determining cerebral death.

Held and Gottstein (182) measured the CBF and $CMRO_2$ in 20 comatose patients. In the 8 patients with irreversible coma who died within 5 days, the $CMRO_2$ was reduced in 3 cases of cerebral death to the point where the O_2 consumption was not measurable. In the other cases the CBF was only slightly decreased and the $CMRO_2$ was 2–3 ml/100g/min. They concluded that a $CMRO_2$ below 1 ml/100g/min may be taken as an indication of a dying or dead brain. Brodersen and Jorgensen (71) concur in this conclusion, stating such a low rate is incompatible with return of consciousness.

Because of the disadvantages and limitations of $CMRO_2$ determinations, increased attention has been given to the chemical measurements of factors that modulate the O_2 consumption—namely, venous oxygen pressure (PvO_2) and differences in the O_2 content of arterial and venous blood—which it was hoped would correlate with $CMRO_2$.

Critical Oxygen Tension.   Most investigators in the last few decades have accepted the conclusions of Opitz and Schneider (357) that the critical level of oxygen tension is approximately a PvO_2 of 19 mm Hg. This was the point at which their animals lost consciousness; death ensued when the PvO_2 reached the range of 12–14 mm Hg. Recently, however, MacMillan and Siesjö (298) have shown in rats that the ability of the brain to withstand anoxic insults is greatly dependent upon the state of cerebral perfusion at the time of the insult. They found that lowering the PvO_2 to 10 mm Hg did not produce significant derangements of cerebral oxidative metabolism provided that the arterial blood pressure and cerebral perfusion pressures were maintained in the normal range. Conversely, Eklöf and Siesjö (128) demonstrated that serious metabolic derangements occurred if the cerebral perfusion was decreased, even though the PvO_2 fell only to 33 mm Hg.

Further evidence that the brain has greater resistance to simple anoxia than previously believed is derived from work by Olsson and Hossmann (356). They showed that cats were able to withstand a long period of anoxia provided the brain was perfused—even with a nonoxygenated electrolyte solution. The accumulation of toxic waste products of cerebral metabolism (such as lactic acid) may be the factor producing irreversible brain unjury, rather than hypoxia per se.

Arteriovenous Oxygen Difference ($AVDO_2$). Although in cerebral death the PvO_2 may be unusually high due to the failure of the brain to take up O_2, the estimates of the differences of the O_2 content of arterial and jugular bulb blood is of more value for the determination of cerebral death than the level of O_2 tension. Theoretically, if, as assumed in cerebral death, there is no CBF, any difference in the O_2 content of arterial and jugular bulb blood should represent extracerebral metabolism. Since this is low in comparison with the high rate of $CMRO_2$, the PvO_2 is high, and the $AVDO_2$ is commonly less than 2 vol %. Paulson et al. (367) have commented upon the high O_2 content of jugular blood in cerebral death. To show that this was due to the external circulation, Minami et al. (322) clamped the external carotid artery and found that the jugular PO_2 dropped to the level of mixed venous blood. Geraud et al. (143) who studied arteriovenous differences of oxygen, glucose, lactate and pyruvate, concluded that the $AVDO_2$ was the most sensitive indicator of brain death; changes in the other metabolic substances were less predictive. Minami et al. found that most cases of cerebral death had an $AVDO_2$ below 3 vol %; in fact, the mean was 1.86 vol %. Bes et al. (48) reported that in 13 cases of deep coma suspected of cerebral death, the $AVDO_2$ was less than 2 vol % in 8 cases and 2–3 vol % in 3 cases, and Brodersen and Jorgensen (71) found such levels in 7 of 11 cases, but they noted that some patients with dead brains had a normal $AVDO_2$ (6 vol %). Again, other comatose patients with luxury perfusion had an $AVDO_2$ under 2 vol %. Although Minami et al. and Yoneda (523) suggest that $AVDO_2$ may be used as a biological test for cerebral death, Brodersen and Jorgensen and Pendl et al. (370) emphasized its unreliability as a predictor of cerebral death.

There is more agreement, however, that the determination of $AVDO_2$ has advantages in differentiating drug induced from other irreversible comas. In barbiturate intoxication, the $AVDO_2$ is normal or increased. This is in line with Sokoloff's report (441) that in severe barbiturate intoxication the $CMRO_2$ is more reduced than the CBF, so that the cerebral O_2 supply is more than adequate.

Lactic Acid Content of the Cerebrospinal Fluid (CSF). Although lactate is increased in the CSF in all cases of coma except barbiturate intoxication, in cerebral death there is an abnormally high lactic acid content (71, 367). Levels from 10.9 to 15.75 mEq/1 (normal = 2 mEq/1) have been reported. The lactate: pyruvate ratio is also increased, and, as might be expected, lactate dehydrogenase is also up. Yashon et al. (521) believe that there is a correlation between the elevated lactic acid levels, the presence of ECS and cerebral death. In this regard, Zattoni et al. (526) have shown that with lactic acid levels of 3.77 mEq/1 the brain is capable of producing potentials having a frequency above 6–7 Hz, whereas when the level of the CSF lactic acid reaches 6.72 mEq/1, as it does in cerebral death, the cerebrum is unable to develop potentials demonstrable with conventional recording.

The metabolic alterations in states of arrested cerebral circulation indicate that the biochemical syndrome of cerebral death consists of the triad of an archaic respiratory quotient, marked drop in the $AVDO_2$ to less than 2 vol %, and an increase in CSF lactic acid to more than 3 mg %. Although $CMRO_2$ changes may occur earlier than angiographic or isotope evidence of circulatory arrest, the technique, even with a mass spectrometer, is complicated; and requiring catheter placements in the jugular bulb and an artery might be hazardous in a patient balanced between life and death.

Chapter VI

Electroencephalographic Findings in Cerebral Death

Introduction

It was natural that the electroencephalogram (EEG) should be chosen as a test for the demonstration of a dead brain, since it is a noninvasive record of brain potentials derived from scalp electrodes. Its undulations provide an objective sign that the cerebrum is active. However, the absence of potential fluctuations in the record does not necessarily justify the conclusion that the brain is no longer functioning. An electroencephalographic tracing (when made under approved recording conditions) that appears to be a straight line has been given various names—flat, isoelectric, null, complete inactivity, electrocerebral silence, electrical silence and absence of biological activity. The American EEG Society's Committee on Cerebral Death (431) recommended "electrocerebral silence" (ECS); the International Federation suggested "electrocerebral inactivity" (11). The synonyms are defined as no electrocerebral activity over two microvolts (μv) when recording from scalp or referential electrode pairs 10 or more centimeters apart with inter-electrode resistances under 10,000 ohms (or impedances under 6,000 ohms) but over 100 ohms. This arbitrary definition does not imply that the brain is not generating any electrical activity, for subcortical or even small cortical discharges of 10μV may be so attenuated that they are not identifiable in the background noise of the recording instrument. Moreover, since in routine electroencephalography the amplification is such that a 50μv signal causes a pen deflection of 7.5 mm or 7.0 μV/mm, any activity under 5μv, which would produce a pen excursion of less than 1 mm, is difficult or impossible to discern. Thus, records described in the EEG literature as "flat" that were recorded at standard gains cannot be accepted as valid evidence of electrocerebral silence. Only when the amplification is such that potentials of 1 to 2 μv give discernible waves in the tracing may an isoelectric record be said to represent an inert brain.

Usually, EEGs on brain death suspects are carried out in intensive care units, recovery rooms or emergency suites where multiple sources of artifact from respirators, monitors, nursing activity, etc., are present. The high amplification required increases the contamination of the record and even meticulous attention to details of technique may not eliminate all artifacts. This poses a problem, for the electroencephalographer must be able to identify all undulations in the record as biological activity or artifacts before he can state that ECS is or is not present.

The artifactual components of an EEG in patients suspected of cerebral death have been discussed by a number of authors (51, 158) and extensively depicted in the *Atlas on Coma and Cerebral Death* (39). The following brief discussion may suffice for the clinician who wishes to know the possible pitfalls and limitation of the EEG in brain death—and yet is not engaged in the actual recording or reading of such EEGs.

The Sources of Artifacts

The electroencephalographer readily recognizes the frequency, wave form and distribution of potentials of cerebral origin; artifacts, however, may mimic brain activity. The timing of such bursts to other events, such as respiration, EKG or the drip of an intravenous infusion may suggest their true nature and source. The adventitious waves arise from (1) the electroencephalograph, (2) the connectors to the patient, (3) the environment and (4) the patient.

The Electroencephalograph.   All amplifying systems generate small potentials—intrinsic noise—which impose a limit on the level of useful amplification of the input potentials. The recommendation of the International Federation of Societies for Electroencephalography and Clinical Neurophysiology requires that with high gain and frequency response and 5,000 ohms across the input, an electroencephalograph should not generate intermittent or transient deflections greater than 2μv once per second.

Electrodes and Electrode Resistances.   The electrodes and their mountings may be responsible for artifacts. Metal disc electrodes may be dislodged or their conducting paste or jelly dry out causing an increased impedance. Needle electrodes inserted into the scalp result in higher resistances that attenuate the electrical signal, in most instruments to an insignificant degree. However, if the resistances of the electrodes are dissimilar, prominent artifacts, usually 60 cycle (line frequency), may be introduced into the EEG channel.

External Sources.   The environment of the patient is responsible for many artifacts. Jarring the bed, the electrode wires or the patient, particularly the head, will produce changes in the potentials. (Figure VI-1).

Feedback or inductance from electrical apparatus used to monitor the patient's vital signs can usually be recognized by the time sequence, and the source verified by temporarily turning off or unplugging the instrument.

Another artifact, often with regular and rhythmic waves time-locked with the respiratory cycle, comes from the respirator, and is due to oscillation of the tubes, movement of the patient's body, or the electrical circuits of the apparatus. It may be eliminated by stopping the respirator briefly. A variety of techniques are used to monitor respiration on the record—an electrode on the patient's chin and another electrode on the respirator apparatus, an accelerometer taped to some part of the respirator, or marking the record manually.

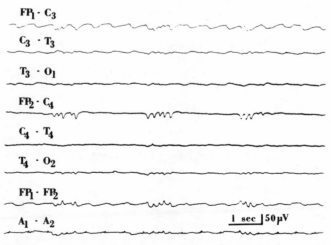

Fig. VI-1. A rhythmic artifact recurring about every three seconds that might be the result of electrical inductance from the respirator or movement of the patient, tubes or electrodes proved to be a ringing telephone (JHH).

The Patient. Potentials generated by the patient are always a possible source of artifact. The artifacts from the heartbeats are usually greater in cases of cerebral death than in routine recording of patients. Their components may be disproportionately large as the result of changes in the EKG due to myocardial infarction or ischemia, the position of the patient's head relative to his body, and the montages used, since the electrical field representation of atrial depolarization (P-wave), ventricular depolarization (QRS) and ventricular repolarization (T-wave) all differ on the scalp (Figure VI-2).

The form of the wave, time-locked to the EKG, usually suggests its identity. The amplitude of the EKG may be decreased by changing the montage to one with less pronounced artifacts. The QRS complex is not the only deflection, for the T-waves at times are prominent. Other rhythmic discharges, time-locked to the QRS complexes and usually ballistocardiographic, are often seen; their artifactual nature and source can be shown by accelerometers.

Methods of eliminating EKG artifact from EEG have been developed, one by using a digital computer, and the other, a more practical method, by analog methods. In the digital method, a template of the EKG appearing in scalp leads (constructed by averaging 200 samples) is subtracted from the EKG-EEG mixture, producing an EKG-free scalp recording composed

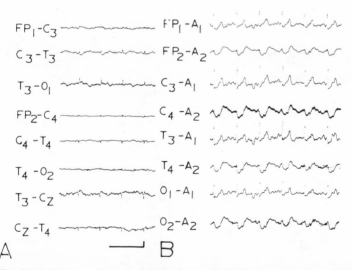

Fig. VI–2. Electrocardiogram artifacts in the EEG (Time scale = 1 second Calibration = 10 μV)

A   Bipolar recording with minimum artifact.
B   Recording with ears as reference leads showing high voltage artifact.

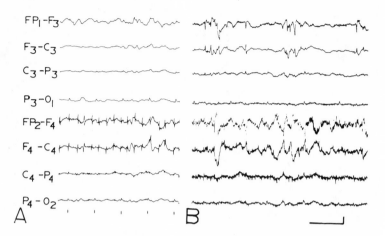

Fig. VI-3,
A Regular spiky muscle artifact in channels 5 and 6. The EKG artifact can be seen in channel 8 and has been indicated at the base.
B Artifacts in channels 1, 2, 5, and 6 are due to eye movements: in channels 5, 6, 7, and 8 are scalp muscle artifacts.

of EEG and system noise. In the analog method, the patient's EKG is sampled from different areas of the neck to obtain the EKG wave form which most closely matches that seen in the EEG; the pure EKG sample is then mixed with the appropriate channel of scalp activity, and the two channels are "subtracted" by means of an operational amplifier, leaving the resulting trace free of EKG artifact.

At times, high amplitude electromyographic potentials generated from scalp or neck muscles may obscure the record and prevent a diagnosis of ECS. EMG potentials usually differ in their frequency distribution from EEG and are recognizable by their high frequency spiking and focal nature. However, they may be sinusoidal, rhythmic and generalized, and not always distinguishable from EEG activity. If they cannot be eliminated by any other means, a muscle relaxant such as succinylcholine (20–40 mg.) or Pavulon®, which produces a longer lasting paralysis, may safely be given intravenously since the patient is already on a respirator (Figure VI-4).

Movements of the orbits generate oculographic potentials (EOG) which can mimic brain waves. Roving eye movements may occur with ECS whenever the cerebral cortex is destroyed leaving the brainstem preserved. By using an analog subtraction technique similar to that used to subtract EKG, the EOG artifact can be eliminated from the EEG record. (51)

Movements of the patient due to decerebrate or decorticate posturing, myoclonic seizures and twitches of various types cause gross artifacts which are usually easily recognized; if necessary, these can be eliminated by the

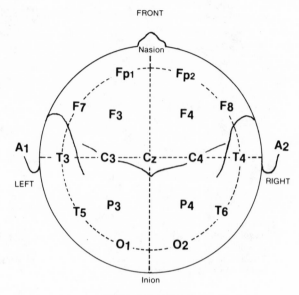

TOP OF HEAD

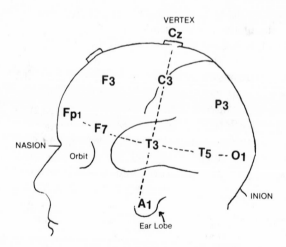

LEFT SIDE OF HEAD

Fig. VI–4. Sketches of the head to show the electrode placements used in the international 10–20 system. For recording in cerebral death suspects, long interelectrode distances are desirable, so the intermediate placements are omitted in some runs and included in others to make the sampling complete.

injection of an anticonvulsant drug such as diazepam. However, a diagnosis of ECS should not be made until the effect of the drug has worn off.

The tongue has a uniform potential gradient from tip to base, the tip being electrically negative relative to the base. Theoretically, glosso-kinetic potentials could obscure electrocerebral silence whenever brainstem function to the level of the pontomedullary junction is intact. Neuromuscular blocking agents may be used in such cases.

Although the frequency of impedance changes in skin potential which accompany sweating are usually less than 0.5 Hz, they may be mistaken for delta activity. Cooling the patient's scalp by applying alcohol between the electrodes may eliminate these potentials.

The most difficult artifacts to eliminate are those resulting from breathing and heartbeat. Head movement caused by respiration or the slight acceleration of the body during ventricular systole (cardioballistographic) can produce potentials which mimic EEG activity. Electrode displacement without head movement can occur if an electrode is placed over a pulsating scalp artery, and produces a characteristic pulse artifact.

An accelerometer on the patient's chest will indicate any movements due to respiration, and will serve as a time reference for artifacts related to pulmonary ventilation (respirator, tubes, electrical contacts, etc.).

Sources of Error in Cerebral Death EEG Records

Both as the result of inadequate knowledge of the medical history or inadequate recording of the EEG, misinterpretations of cerebral death records may occur either in the direction of falsely diagnosing ECS or falsely asserting biological activity. These errors may be avoided if certain basic rules are followed.

False Positives in EEG Diagnosis. A number of conditions may produce ECS of a temporary nature. Certain new anesthetic agents may induce cerebral silence, although evoked potentials can still be elicited. Hypothermia below 28° C may be associated with a reversible ECS. A number of other conditions may cause a temporary ECS in a clinic setting. The technical factors that may give a false picture of ECS occur at three levels, (1) the patient-electrode interface, (2) the electroencephalograph, and (3) the sampling of the EEG.

Potential Technical Factors in the False Diagnosis of ECS

Faulty Electrode Placement.   An insufficiently wide distribution of electrodes may lead to misdiagnosis of ECS if the absence of EEG activity is widespread but not complete.

Short interelectrode distance.   This can result in failure to detect very low voltage activity which, with greater interelectrode distances, might be apparent. The potential difference between electrodes is proportional to the square of the interelectrode distance up to about 10 cm. The American Electroencephalographic Society recommends minimal interelectrode distances of 10 cm, which is about double that of the conventional 10-20 system (Figure VI-4).

Very High or Very Low Interelectrode Impedances.   Very low impedances, essentially a short circuit, would give an isopotential tracing regardless of the true interelectrode potential. Very high impedances attenuate brain waves and can make low voltage records appear flat.

Errors in Amplification and Recording

At the machine level, several factors may contribute to a false diagnosis of ECS.

Failure to Record at Sufficiently High Gains.   At the standard gain of 7.5 μV/mm, a 2μv signal will produce a pen displacement that can not be detected by the human eye. Using increased sensitivity (at least 2.0 μV/mm) during part of the recording, it is possible to see deflections that would just exceed the minimal standards for ECS. Of course EKG potentials and the system noise are enhanced to an equal extent and may still exceed 2 μv.

Short Time Constants.   A pseudo-isoelectric recording may result from short time constants if the existing EEG activity is of a very low voltage and frequency; for example, standard time constants between 0.1 and 0.2 seconds would attenuate a 5μv. 1 Hz sinusoidal rhythm to 0.4–1.4 μv, which could not be identified in the noise of the system. The American

Electroencephalographic Society's recommendation for the use of time constants of 0.3–0.4 seconds would increase the recorded amplitude of the 5μv. 1 Hz activity to 2.2–2.7μv, which would just be seen if not obscured by slow wave artifacts from respiration.

Short Circuiting of Current.   At the jackbox, cable or machine, a short circuit could lead to a false isopotential record despite the proper application of electrodes and calibration of the channels. As a precaution, each electrode of the montage should be touched with a pencil point to create an artifact potential in the record when a silent EEG is first recorded if EKG or other artifactual material is not already present.

Inadequate Sampling of the EEG.   Failure to test for electrical reactivity to visual, auditory and other sensory stimuli; one of these modalities may give a response when the others do not.

Inadequate Length of Recording.   Periods of electrical silence and burst suppression phenomena are seen following many CNS insults; a minimum recording time of 30 minutes is necessary to establish the absence of such periodic activity.

Because the maximal revival time of the EEG following some CNS insults is not known for man, and because the level of EEG activity in coma, especially if complicated by drugs, may fluctuate considerably and show marked periodicity, a number of serial records may be desirable in some cases.

False Negatives in EEGs

Electrical Artifacts of Biological Origin.   Although a false positive diagnosis of electrocerebral silence is potentially a more serious error, the converse situation may occur as a consequence of numerous extracranial generators of electrical potentials such as the heart, eyes, tongue and muscle. Foremost among the extracranial contributions to the EEG is the electrocardiogram, which Gaches et al. (141) found to contaminate more than half of the EEGs. The EKG potentials in low voltage records are frequently the dominant wave form and may mask EEG slow wave activity that is less than 25% of the amplitude of the QRS complex. Probably the EKG activity in about one-third of the cases with isoelectric records is of sufficient amplitude to obscure significant EEG activity.

Computerized Techniques for EEG Recording in Cerebral Death

Preliminary studies have indicated that computer techniques may simplify the reading of EEG records of individuals suspected of cerebral death. The computer has been used for elimination of extraneous material in EEGs, condensation of EEG data, and analysis of frequency and power.

Synthetic EEG Records. The recognition of biological activity in the presence of extraneous activity such as EKG, instrument noise or muscle potentials is difficult if not impossible. To determine the ability of the human eye to recognize biological activity in a background of noise and EKG, Bickford et al. (51) synthesized, by means of a computer, a series of records with varying amounts of each of the above ingredients. Even the most astute clinical electroencephalographers were unable to detect EEG activity of only 2 μv (peak-to-peak amplitude) in the presence of amounts of EKG and background noise commonly encountered in cerebral death records. In fact, the EEG activity had to exceed this amplitude by a factor of 2 or 3 to be identifiable in the traces. It is difficult for an electroencephalographer to identify 2 μv peak-to-peak amplitude EEG activity in a background either of 10 μv EMG or of EKG and background noise. With background activity of higher amplitude, the difficulties are accentuated. In fact, the current requirement by the American Electroencephalographic Society for an isoelectric trace—no evidence of EEG activity above 2 μv— may be beyond the reader's visual ability (51).

Compressed Spectral Analysis (CSA). In order to apply computerized techniques to the EEG write-out, it is necessary to transfer the traces to tape. Conventional EEG recordings may be converted back into electrical form for appropriate computer display and analysis using the Barlow-Shipton optical scanner. The faithful reproduction of the reconstituted trace may be controlled by its printout, which must be indistinguishable on visual inspection from the original ink-written trace, and by spectral analyses of the original data from the magnetic tape and the curve-written data input, which should not differ in their profiles by more than 10% (51).

With this converted EEG, a number of computer-processed analyses are possible. The Expanded Low Frequency Compression Spectral Analysis is a frequency distribution that is more appropriate for the coma record than the conventional 0.25–16 Hz displays used in clinical CSAs in which the cyclic EEG changes in coma frequently are not well displayed.

The CSA technique of EEG analysis is one way to overcome the problem of EMG artifact. Because of the randomness in the frequency of EMG potentials, little power is generated in any given frequency (51). For this reason, sustained muscle contractions introduce little artifact into CSAs and intermittent contractions such as facial twitching result in only a slow wave artifact that does not obscure activity at other frequencies.

EKG Subtraction.   One difficulty in making a decision of ECS is the presence of relatively high amplitude EKG artifacts, especially if there is a prominent T-wave component that may mask low-voltage EEG activity.

With simple instrumentation, one can subtract the EKG artifact and leave the remaining slow waves to be quantified by voltage integration. With such quantitative data, the electroencephalographer can come to a rational opinion concerning the existence of isopotentiality or electrocerebral silence. The technique consists of a simple nulling method that samples the EKG from an appropriate position on the neck, subtracts it from the trace containing EKG and then integrates the remaining activity by means of an operational amplifier. The result appears as pulses on a channel of the EEG and can be read off in microvolts by counting the number of pulses per page.

Bickford (51) believes that electroencephalographers should speak in terms of recorded activity in microvolts instead of electrocerebral silence. Even with good techniques the noise level is frequently of the order of 2–3 μv which approaches the level of activity required for electrocerebral silence (2 μv).

In clinical practice, computerized techniques available for the elimination of EKG artifacts and for the estimation of the amount of artifactual or biological material in the record are rarely used. In the usual case, elaborate computer techniques are unnecessary, but in cases with artifact and low voltage activity that may be biological, the printout may demonstrate activity that is not apparent on visual inspection. However, not all cyclic activity shown by the computerized analysis is biological; rhythmically recurrent artifacts will be treated by the computer the same as biological data.

Electroencephalographic Recording in Patients Suspected of Cerebral Death

Because the results of EEG are so significant in making a final confirmation of cerebral death, and since the recording must often be done in rooms without shielding, with many electrical appliances in operation and with doctors and nurses moving about, the technical aspects of obtaining a record are important considerations. The American EEG Society has given a great deal of critical thought to determining the best montage, the means of applying electrodes, and the recording of the traces (11). Considering the difficulties that are encountered in recording in unshielded areas such as emergency rooms, operating theaters, intensive care units, recovery suites and wards, they have recommended the following:

1. A minimum of eight scalp electrodes and ear reference electrodes
2. Interelectrode resistances under 10,000 ohms but over 100 ohms
3. Test of integrity of recording system by deliberate creation of electrode artifact by manipulation
4. Interelectrode distances of at least 10 cm
5. Gains increased during most of the recording from 7.0µV to 2.0µV/mm
6. The use of 0.3 or 0.4 sec time constants during part of the recording
7. Recording with an EKG and other monitoring devices such as a pair of electrodes on the dorsum of the right hand to detect extra-cerebral potentials
8. Tests for reactivity to pain, loud noises or light
9. A 30-minute total recording time
10. Recording by a qualified technician
11. Repeating the record if the ECS is doubtful
12. Telephone transmitted EEGs are not appropriate for determination of ECS.

The recommendations of the American EEG Society regarding the number of electrodes as well as their placements (10-20 system) have proved satisfactory. Interelectrode distances of 10 cm are recommended by the American EEG Society but some electroencephalographers (EEGers) suggest that 8 cm might be more appropriate. Both bipolar and monopolar montages are desirable. An noncephalic (2-electrode) lead on the dorsum of the right hand for control of muscle "noise" may be put in the first channel and lead one EKG in the second channel. Minimal montages or runs in the other six channels are:

1. Fp2-C4, C4-O2, Fpl-C3, C3-O1, T4-Cz, Cz-T3;
2. F8-T6, T6-T5, T5-F7, F7-F8, F4-P4, F3-P3;
3. F4-A1, C4-A1, O2-A1, F3-A2, C3-A2, O1-A2;
4. Fp2-Cz, F8-Cz, T6-Cz, Fpl-Cz, F7-Cx, T5-Cz;
5. Fp2-T4, T4-O2, Fpl-T3, T3-O1, P4-A1, P3-A2.

Time constants of 0.3 or 0.4 seconds are desirable and, if necessary, 35 or 75 Hz filters may be used. Cutaneous pinpricks to the extremities as well as auditory and photic stimuli should be applied while the record is being watched for evoked potentials. An ideal study is continued for 30 minutes, during which, if the traces appear to be isoelectric, the gains should be at 2μV/mm for approximately 20 minutes. A number of devices have been suggested to confirm that the electroencephalograph is operating properly. Some homely maneuvers—inserting EKG in the record, jiggling the lead wires and introducing 60 cycle—will serve essentially the same purpose.

Electrodes and Electrode Resistances. Various types of electrodes and mountings are used in clinical electroencephalography. The ideal goal is a stable low resistance (or impedance) contact with the patient's skin, which probably is best accomplished by metal disc electrodes and a conducting paste or jelly with collodion as an adherent to the scalp. Because electrodes must be applied under less than optimal conditions, some electroencephalographers prefer to insert needle electrodes into the scalp and hold them in place with strips of adhesive tape. Even though these electrodes have a higher resistance than discs, the records usually are satisfactory.

The American EEG Committee on Cerebral Death has recommended that the resistance between electrodes should be 100 to 10,000 ohms. High resistance electrodes attenuate the electrical signal, but in most instruments to an insignificant degree. However, the resistances of the electrodes should be similar since the EEG amplifiers are sensitive to differences in the electrode resistances of their imput. Prominent artifacts, particularly of 60 cycle (line frequency), are commonly due to high impedance in one of the electrodes to the involved channel.

Line frequency artifacts appearing in all channels are usually due to inadequate grounding. If this is the case, a separate ground connection to a cold water pipe should resolve the difficulty.

The Interpretation of the EEG

The EEG examination on a patient suspected of cerebral death is usually requested when resuscitative measures have been exhausted. These therapeutic procedures may take from a few hours to several days. In hospitals where an active transplant service is seeking donor organs, pressure may be applied to speed up the therapeutic endeavors so that the patient may be declared cerebrally dead before cardiac arrest and the deterioration of organs can occur. In some cases, the attending physician, aware of the irreparable damage to the brain and the futility of therapeutic measures, may accept the inevitable and stop unusual therapeutic measures without waiting for clinical and laboratory evidence of cerebral death. However, especially when requests are made in the middle of the night, the EEG examination may be delayed a few hours by these resuscitative efforts and by the inability of a technician to reach the hospital. In the Collaborative Study, the EEG examinations were performed an average of 8.4 hours after the initiation of artificial respiration (Table VI-1). This allowed time for cardiovascular resuscitation and pulmonary care to improve the patient's general condition. The first EEG recording should not be done in the initial shock stage, but during a stabilized state, especially if certification of cerebral death is being considered, for shock can reduce the cerebral perfusion pressure and temporarily depress the EEG. Although somewhat neglected in the past, this is an important consideration in cardiac disease where shock may in fact be responsible for coma and apnea.

Since the electroencephalograms are examined not for wave form or frequency, but for the absence of any electrical activity arising from the brain, some consideration should be given to the characteristics of such a record.

Isoelectric (Flat) Electroencephalogram

In the past, the term "flat electroencephalogram" has been used with various connotations. A low voltage record that may occasionally be encountered in normal subjects has been termed flat. Other abnormal traces made at standard gains with almost imperceptible undulations, which at high amplification would have shown waves of 5 to 10 μV, have also been called flat. Only in the past decade have electroencephalographers fol-

Table VI-1. Elapsed Time Between Beginning Artificial Respiration or Apnea, Whichever Was Later, and the Start of the Initial EEG.

Elapsed Time (hours)	Total Number of Cases
0–0.9	27
1–1.9	48
2–2.9	53
3–3.9	45
4–4.9	30
5–11.9	103
12+	186
Unknown or no EEG	11
Total	503

lowed the requirements of the American EEG Society's Committee on Cerebral Death for recording on patients suspected of having a dead brain (431) and reserved the term flat or electrocerebral silence (ECS) for a trace with no activity over $2\mu V$ recorded at a gain of at least $2\mu V = 1$ mm (about the upper limit of most electroencephalographs).

In the past, flat records have been reported in a number of conditions—postictal coma, anesthesia, sedative drug intoxications, encephalitis, hypothermia and cerebral trauma. Because of the earlier use of this term to denote a low voltage record, it is advisable to review these cases in order to assess their validity according to current standards.

The largest survey of flat electroencephalograms was carried out in 1969 by the American EEG Society's Ad Hoc Committee on EEG Criteria for the Determination of Cerebral Death (431). Of 1,665 patients with records pronounced flat by 100 reporting members of the American EEG Society, only seven persons recovered; three had sedative drug intoxication, one insulin coma, one asphyxia from drowning, one cardiac arrest and one circulatory collapse during an operation. However, the only records in which the Committee concurred in the diagnosis of ECS were those of the three poisoning cases. The others were considered to have low-voltage activity or were unavailable for examination.

Postictal Coma.   Immediately after spontaneous or traumatic cerebral accidents, especially if they are associated with shock and a low perfusion pressure, the electroencephalogram may be isoelectric. Pampiglione and Harden (365) state "a transitory EEG equipotentiality is common immediately after cerebral ischemia or anoxia, a cerebral contusion, or after administration of some drugs. However, in the context of resuscitation after circulatory arrest (i.e., excluding head injuries and poisoning) whenever equipotentiality persisted for over 2–3 hours at normothermia with satisfactory circulatory and respiratory conditions, no phase activity ever returned."

Yet, Bushart and Rittmeyer (81) reported a patient with cardiac arrest who had ECS for 2 days with recovery. He had no intoxication but his neurological status during and subsequent to the isoelectric record is not given. Schwartz (420) mentioned a 38-year-old woman suffering from multiple sclerosis and epilepsy who was admitted to the hospital in a terminal postictal coma. Unfortunately, the patient's temperature and blood pressure were not given, so that the significance of the reported nonexistent or imperceptible EEG activity is not apparent.

Anesthesia.   In the lower stage of anesthesia, especially if some of the new agents have been administered, the EEG may be isoelectric, even when high gains are used. However, these states are induced under controlled conditions so that the isoelectric record is a temporary effect, and would not be confused with a permanent loss of cerebral potentials.

Sedative Drug Intoxications. Numerous cases of drug coma have been reported with flat electroencephalograms. Most of these reports appeared before rigid requirements for an isoelectric record were accepted, and, accordingly, few of the published traces would meet current standards for ECS. However, it must be admitted that competent EEGers read these records as isoelectric, and even if later reviewers would not concur in the opinion, these readings must be accepted as meeting the standard of that time. For this reason, consideration must be given to the usual and customary interpretations of EEGs that may not attain research standards.

In cases of drug intoxication, the neurological depression may be of such a degree that the clinical signs of cerebral death are met—except, perhaps, the dilated pupils that most sedative drugs (the notable exceptions being glutethimide and scopolamine) do not produce (Figure VI–5). The neurological depression and isoelectric EEG may last more than 24 hours and yet the patient may recover (55, 169, 221, 247). With effective treatment such as dialysis, the EEG develops slow potentials and the coma lightens in a few hours. However, not all drugs, even in toxic amounts, cause ECS. Powner (381) lists phenothiazines, atropine, tricyclic antidepressants, nitrazepam, salicylates, heroin, glutethimide, insecticides and amanita phalloides (mushroom poisoning) as drugs that often do not depress the EEG. The more common sedatives producing ECS include barbiturates, methaqualone, diazepam, mecloqualone, meprobamate and trichloroethylene.

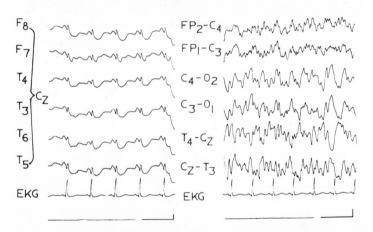

Fig. VI–5. Tracings taken during drug-induced ECS (A) and about 24 hours after (B) dialysis showing high-voltage slow activity. The patient's record became normal in 3 days. (time scale = 1 second calibration = 50 μV).

Of course, any drug that depresses respiration so that apnea develops may be associated with an anoxic encephalopathy and ECS.

The confirmatory tests for cerebral death are important in cases suspected of drug intoxication, for unless there has been a complicating anoxic episode, the $AVDO_2$ is high, the CBF is unimpaired, and the $CMRO_2$ is within normal limits.

Cortical Death.   Comatose patients with intact brainstem functions may have isoelectric EEGs. This condition has been termed cortical or neocortical death. Two cases with pathological studies of the brain were reported by Brierley et al. (67). In the *Atlas of EEG in Coma and Brain Death* (39), cases V-9 and V-10 illustrate the EEG findings. Neither of these cases met clinical criteria for cerebral death and even the diagnosis of ECS was questionable. A number of other cases reported under various titles are to some degree similar (40, 66, 106, 206, 218, 297). Jonkman (220) reported a 2-year-old child with encephalitis who had electrocerebral silence but intact brainstem reflexes. In this case, a depth recording demonstrated subcortical activity. Visser (484) referred briefly to a 76-year-old comatose woman with ECS who breathed spontaneously.

It is apparent that although ECS in any record is a serious omen, the absence of electrical potentials is not necessarily indicative of either total cerebral dysfunction or a dead brain.

The Electroencephalogram in Cerebral Death Suspects

The electrical potentials in comatose and apneic persons may exhibit great variations, from a tracing that appears practically normal (alpha coma) or a greatly disorganized record to one with complete absence of all discernible activity. These alterations are described in atlases of electroencephalography, and their relations to a dead brain require only brief comment.

The most common finding in comatose and apneic patients is probably a localized or generalized slowing of the predominant rhythm (Figure VI–6). This delta or theta activity may be constantly present or it may be intermittent with relatively normal frequencies between the slow waves. Not infrequently, the slow waves have faster activity superimposed (Figure VI–7). In some records, bursts of high-amplitude theta activity occur locally or throughout the head with practically no discernible potentials in the intervals, which usually last just a few seconds (Figure VI–8). The slow

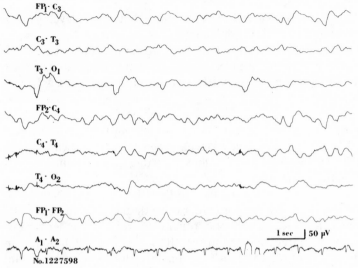

Fig. VI–6. Record taken at normal gains on a comatose and apneic patient who had been on the respirator about 24 hours. There is slow, irregular activity of varying frequency in all leads. (JHH)

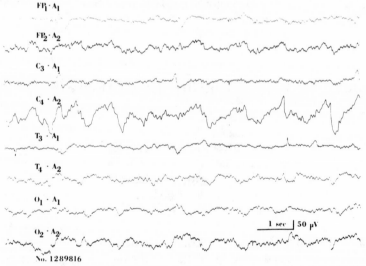

Fig. VI–7. Record from a comatose and apneic patient, in which there is alpha and beta activity superimposed upon background slowing of varying potential. (JHH)

activity or bursts may be associated with spikes, although a typical spike and wave pattern is rarely seen. Occasionally the spiky activity occurs once or twice a second with no intervening waves (Figure VI–9).

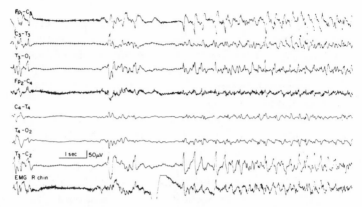

Fig. VI–8. Supression bursts in a patient comatose and apneic as the result of a head injury. Note the episodic clusters of sharp waves in all channels with almost a flat record between the bursts. (JHH)

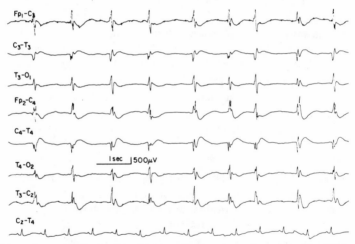

Fig. VI–9. Fairly regular generalized spiking in a comatose and apneic patient. The EKG seen in channel 8 is not time-related to the artifacts. (JHH)

The pattern of the EEG may be related in part to the underlying condition responsible for the coma. Depressant drugs are likely to cause generalized slowing, although initially fast beta activity may be seen in barbiturate intoxication. Liver disease is frequently associated with triphasic activity and renal disorders with slow waves. Intracranial lesions may produce localized abnormalities and asymmetrics. Trauma to the head may be associated with focal or generalized alterations. When intracranial hypertension has increased to the point of eliminating cerebral blood flow, the EEG potentials are likely to be generally depressed and slow. In general, the initial EEG findings are not reliable prognosticators of the later developments—either clinical or electroencephalographic. As mentioned previously, many factors, some systemic and some neurological, influence the outcome.

Insofar as the diagnosis of cerebral death is concerned, the interpretation of the electroencephalogram need only be categorized as (1) the presence of activity of neuronal origin (biological activity), (2) the absence of potentials of neuronal origin (electrocerebral silence), or (3) equivocal findings (artifactual obscuration of the record so that a definitive diagnosis is not possible). Since the identification of a dead brain and not a prognostication of the quality of surviving life is the goal, this simple classification is adequate. On that basis, in the Collaborative Study the records were classified as ECS in 187 cases, as biological activity in 283 (100 later developed a flat record before death) and as equivocal in 30 cases (Table VI–2). Although 188 records were considered to have artifacts confusing the interpretations to some extent, a diagnosis on the initial EEG was possible in all but 30 cases. In 19 cases, the records were judged not to meet the standards of the American EEG Society, usually because the period of recording was too short. Although many records had muscle artifacts, they were sufficiently troublesome that relaxants had to be given in only 34 cases. Probably a diagnosis of ECS would have been possible if such drugs had been used in more patients with equivocal records (Figure VI–10).

Equivocal Records.   No matter how meticulous the recording, a few traces will be unclassifiable because of artifacts or undiagnosible waves in the records. Such adventitious activity does not prevent a positive interpretation if one or more artifact-free segments of the record have unquestionable biological activity. However, any persistent unidentifiable baseline undulations preclude a diagnosis of ECS, and such records, the majority of which are probably isoelectric, must be classified as equivocal. In the Collaborative Study, the 30 records so diagnosed on the initial

Table VI–2.   Results of the Initial EEG.

Findings	Total Number of Cases		
	yes	no	Not done
Technically Satisfactory	458	42	3
ECS	187	313	3
Equivocal	188	312	3
Biological Activity	283	217	3

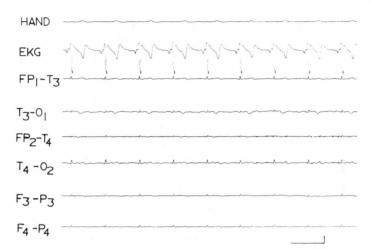

Fig. VI–10. Electrocerebral silence in a head-injured man. The first channel from electrodes on the dorsum of the hand shows the inherent noise. The second is the EKG, and the remainder show no activity except artifacts time-locked with the EKG. (time scale = 1 second calibration = 10 μV) (JHH)

examination represent only a small fraction (16%) of the tracings that had complicating artifactual material.

The Accuracy of Reader Interpretation. The accuracy of the readings has been a moot point. In the Collaborative Study all records were reviewed by the project coordinator. Records of questionable interpretation or of special interest, approximately 15% of the total, were referred to a panel of senior electroencephalographer consultants. If the readings of the local EEGers and the project coordinator agreed, it was assumed that further review by the panel would also produce concordance. On the basis of these checks by the coordinator and the review panel, which disagreed with the primary reader in only 13 cases, it seems probable that had the entire 500 cases been reviewed by the EEG consultants, the lack of concord would have been less than 3%. It should be noted that the panel judged only 6 initial EEGs read as ECS to have had biological activity.

The Course of the EEG in the Evolution of Cerebral Death

Knowledge of the changing electrical activity of the brain as the result of a progressive cerebral death is incomplete because of the technical difficulties of recording during the early postictal period. In the Collaborative Study, only 218 patients had EEGs made within the first 6 hours after meeting the entrance requirements; of these persons, 80 had ECS. In the first 12 hours, 306 EEGs were done, and of these 126 had ECS (Table VI-3). After 24 hours the number of persons having ECS in their initial records decreases; persons who have their first inactive tracing after 4 days are rarely alive in 24 hours to have a second record. Thus, approximately 38% of the patients developing ECS in the first two days will have iso-electric records 24 hours later, but thereafter few patients live long enough to have multiple inactive traces. Although the electroencephalograms may change from biological activity to ECS at any time, after a week the chances are slight that such an alteration, except as an agonal event, will occur.

Transition from Biological Activity to ECS. Approximately 40% of apneic and comatose patients have ECS in their initial records; another 22% will develop flat records over a period of several days. It was hoped that the characteristics of the initial EEG abnormalities might indicate the future occurrence of ECS. However, probably because of a number of factors—the different primary disorders, the varying sites of cerebral pathology, and the cause of the progression (aggravation of the primary condition, secondary edema or extracranial factors such as circulatory failure)—the

Table VI-3.   Relationship of Single and 24 Hour ECS to Time in Study.

Time of ECS After Entry Into Study (hours)	ECS	
	single flat record (cases)	flat record with 2nd ECS in 24 or more hours (cases)
<6	43	37
6–12	29	17
12–24	48	18
24–48	27	16
48–72	16	6
72–96	8	4
96–120	5	—
120–144	1	—
144–168	4	—
168–336	3	1
>336	1	—
Unknown	2	1

There were 43 cases with a single flat EEG within 6 hours of eligibility (entry) to study. In addition, there were 37 cases with a flat EEG within 6 hours of eligibility to study, all of whom had a second flat EEG in 24 or more hours.
Between 6 and 11.9 hours after eligibility, 29 cases for the first time had a single flat record and 17 additional cases for the first time had a flat record with a second flat EEG in 24 or more hours.

initial electroencephalographic pattern proved not to be predictive of ECS. Mutuskina (340) also noted that although the wave form of the initial EEG gave some idea of the extent of brain damage, its morphology was not a reliable indicator of the outcome. Perhaps a better predictive index might be obtained with the visual assessment and coding of the 51 variables, 49 of which related to EEG, that Binnie et al. (52) described. It is uncertain whether this method could be successfully applied to brain death cases, which require predictions within hours of their ictus, since Binnie et al.'s EEGs were made a few days to a week after resuscitation.

The transition from an active to a flat EEG may be gradual or sudden, the latter probably due to collapse of the cardiovascular system. In the *Atlas of Coma and Cerebral Death* (39) examples of both types of transition are shown (*Atlas*, Fig. V–1 to V–5). Rarely is the exact moment of transition recorded by electroencephalography, so that the frequency of these two types is unknown. However, when arterial hypotension precipitates the flat record, the activity may return if the blood pressure is increased by speeding up the injection of a vasopressor agent. On occasion, ECS has been seen to come and go as the pressure fell and rose.

The Return of Biological Activity.   Brain damage from whatever cause is usually permanent, but some pharmacological agents and endogenous intoxications have only a temporary depressing or paralyzing effect on neuronal activity (Figure VI–5). Many cases of coma due to sedative drugs have been reported to have isoelectric EEGs that have subsequently returned to normal as the coma receded (55, 221, 415). Moreover, a few patients deeply unconscious from other causes with isoelectric records have regained biological activity. Leenstra-Borsje (280) reported 2 cases with ECS who developed electrical activity after 7 hours and 2 days; however, both patients died. In general, once an electroencephalogram has become isoelectric, unless systemic etiological factors—intoxication, hypopiesis or hypothermia—can be corrected, the chances are slight that biological activity will recur. In some cases, artifactual material may obscure neuronal potentials so that a spurious impression of an isoelectric record is given; subsequent records with unequivocal activity may suggest a return of biological activity. In the Collaborative Study series, 7 patients were considered to have electrocerebral silence in one record and in subsequent records to have biological activity; three of these patients, two of whom survived, had exogenous intoxications. A review of the traces of the other cases raised the question whether in the initial records artifactual material might have been obscuring biological activity. However, there is no doubt that competent EEGers will occasionally encounter such cases and interpret them, probably correctly, as restitution of biological activity.

Bennett (38) notes that this is likely to occur when the initial record is made shortly after the ictus. In such cases, cardiovascular shock may be the cause of the isoelectric electroencephalogram. *The Atlas of Coma and Cerebral Death* (39) gives several illustrations (*Atlas* cases V–6 and V–7) of the recovery from ECS. The biological activity returns with intermittent or continuous slow baseline swings. These slow (1 Hz), low undulations, sometimes in bursts, gradually become more complex with faster frequencies superimposed, until in 3 to 5 days the slower activity drops out leaving a relatively normal alpha record. *Atlas* case V–8 illustrates the initial depression of cerebral activity after a cardiorespiratory arrest. This patient did not meet criteria of cerebral death in that the pupillary reflexes were sluggish and there was evidence of cerebral blood flow. The blood pressure at the time of the EEG is not given.

Correlation of EEG and Clinical Findings

There is no doubt that the EEG findings correlate with a number of clinical factors found in patients suspected of cerebral death. To some extent, they relate to the time on the respirator—the longer the ventilation, the higher the proportion of ECS records.

Correlation with Primary Diagnosis.   In the Collaborative Study, the EEG findings correlated with many of the primary diagnoses. Absence of biological activity was high in cerebral neoplasms (65% of the brain tumor patients had ECS), CNS infections (60%), trauma (55%) and subarachnoid hemorrage (54%); in other diagnostic categories, the incidence of absence of biological activity was lower—cerebral thrombosis (36%), metabolic disorders (27%), cardiac disturbances (24%), cerebral embolism (16%) and intoxication (9%).

Correlation with Outcome.   All observers have noted that the EEG activity had a high correlation with survival, and a negative correlation with death. The presence of any biological activity in the EEG was a favorable omen, for of 241 patients with biological activity in the initial record, 42 survived, whereas of 187 with ECS in the initial record only 2—both drug cases—lived. Even in moribund patients, the presence of biological activity was associated with a prolonged existence, in some cases to more than four weeks, whereas cases with ECS were dead within a week of the first flat record. The high mortality associated with ECS is apparent within the first 24 hours, for by this time 43% of the cases with initial ECS have been declared dead (Table VI–4), and within 24 hours of the first ECS on any record 51% have been pronounced dead, some as cerebrally dead. If biological activity is present in the initial record, less than 25% of the patients die within 24 hours (Table VI–5); of those cases with records diagnosed as equivocal, 30% are dead within the first day.

Correlation with Clinical Cerebral Death. In those individuals who meet criteria of brain death in which electroencephalography is not a mandatory requirement, it is of interest to note the state of the cerebral electrical activity. Based upon the findings of the Collaborative Study, from 8% to 40% of persons meeting different sets of clinical criteria for brain death

Table VI–4.   Relationship of Time of Death From Entrance to EEG Findings.

	Initial Biological Activity	Initial ECS		
		All Cases	Cerebral* Death	Cardiac Death
Elapsed Time	No. of Cases	No. of Cases	No. of Cases	No. of Cases
<1 hour	1	1	0	1
1–5.9	15	30	6	24
6–11.9	15	15	5	10
12–23.9	23	34	14	20
1–1.9 days	56	77	45	32
2–2.9	37	15	4	11
3–3.9	24	6	0	6
4–6.9	27	7	1	6
1–1.9 weeks	21			
2–3.9	13			
>4 weeks	9			
Total	241	185	75	110

*Resuscitative efforts stopped

Table VI–5.   Time of Death After First ECS.

Time (Hours)	Number alive at beginning of interval
0–1	287
1–6	281
6–12	234
12–24	208
24–48	140
48–72	42
72–96	21
96–168	15
168–336	1

had biological activity in their electroencephalograms. Powner and Fromm (382) report that 14% of patients referred for EEGs with a diagnosis of cerebral death did not have isoelectric records. However, since all cases died, they concluded that the EEG findings of neuronal activity did not predict a favorable outcome, and hence, they question that an isoelectric EEG should be a mandatory requirement for the determination of cerebral death. Obviously, the question is whether the criteria of cerebral death should identify a dead or a moribund brain.

Correlation with Neuropathological Findings. The EEG and neuropathological findings often correlate. In the Collaborative Study (99) patients with biological activity in the last EEG had fewer swollen brains, fewer cerebral herniations and fewer respirator brains than those with ECS. The location of the lesions was not a significant determinant of a flat EEG, since the percentage of patients with brainstem lesions having ECS was approximately the same (63%) as those with diffuse cerebral lesions (60%) or focal cortical lesions (62%). However, biological activity in the EEG had a better but negative correlation with a respirator brain than did ECS. Although one might expect that the EEG would be flat if the neuropathological diagnosis was respiratory brain, a few patients considered to have respirator brains had biological activity in their last EEG within an hour or so of death.

Correlation with Cephalic Reflexes. Although cephalic reflexes are mediated through the brainstem and the EEG is predominantly related to cortical activity, there is a fairly close correlation between the activity of the two. At the initial examination, moribund persons with a flat EEG had absence of pupillary, corneal and oculocephalic reflexes in 99% of cases; of vestibular, audio-ocular, snout and jaw reflexes in 97% of cases; of pharyngeal, swallowing and cough reflexes in 85% of cases; and of all cephalic reflexes in 78% (Table VI–6). This relationship persisted as time passed and some persons had cardiac arrest. However, pharyngeal, cough and swallowing reflexes tended to persist several days after the other cephalic reflexes had disappeared in the surviving persons. The spinal reflexes, as might be expected, were present even longer in the few lingering patients. Hence, there is some variation in the vulnerability and survival of the individual cephalic reflexes.

This variability of the individual reflexes may be demonstrated by an analysis of the relationship of the presence or absence of each cephalic reflex and the state of the EEG (Table VI–7). The correlation between absence of all cephalic reflex activity and ECS is very high; the association is equally strong between the pupillary reflex and the EEG. Except for the audio-ocular and snout reflexes, the absence of other cephalic reflexes

Table VI–6. Time of Disappearance of Reflexes in Moribund Persons With ECS.

	Time After Entry (Hours)										
	0	6	12	24	48	72	96	120	144	168	>192
No. of cases examined	172	175	165	132	63	35	26	18	6	4	2
Reflex						No. absent					
Pupillary	171	173	164	131	all						
Corneal	171	174	164	131	all						
Oculocephalic	171	174	164	131	all						
Vestibular	166	170	161	127	all						
Audio-ocular	169	172	164	130	all						
Snout	166	170	161	127	all						
Pharyngeal	148	152	152	117	61	all					
Swallowing	144	151	161	118	61	33	25	17	all		
Cough	150	152	151	120	61	33	all				
Jaw Jerk	165	169	161	128	all						
All cephalic	135	143	144	114	61	32	24	17	all		
Tendon	101	87	83	66	33	16	16	8	3	2	all
Muscle tone	141	141	144	116	57	31	24	16	all		
Plantar	118	131	122	83	47	27	21	16	4	3	all
Induced movements	142	147	135	98	50	27	20	15	4	2	all

has a strong correlation with ECS. However, there is no absolute relationship between absence of biological EEG activity and any cephalic areflexia.

Depth Recording

Recording from the brain substance by means of depth electrodes is not simple because of the artifacts introduced by resuscitative equipment and local encephalic instability. Nevertheless, the surface ECS is confirmed although occasionally in the majority of cases, activity may be present in subcortical ganglia such as the thalamus when the scalp records are flat. The technique might be used as a confirmatory test when a very early statement regarding death is required.

Findji et al. (134) studied ten patients in deep and irreversible coma with depth recordings. A nine-pole electrode was inserted through a frontal burr hole in nine cases, and in the tenth case two bipolar stereotaxic electrodes were introduced into the thalamic structures of both sides. In two of three cases in irreversible coma, no activity was found at any level. In the third case, 24 hours after respiratory arrest, 1–2 per second slow waves of about 10–20 µv amplitude were seen. In the other 7 cases, electrical activity was present at all levels, including the scalp. The tenth case,

Table VI–7.   Relationship of Cephalic Reflexes to ECS.

Reflexes	ECS	Not ECS	Total	X^2	p
All Cephalic					
Absent	209	72	281	106.11	<0.001
Present	43	132	175		
Total	252	204	456		
Pupillary					
Absent	272	112	384	117.8	<0.001
Present	16	101	117		
Total	288	213	501		
Oculocephalic					
Absent	276	156	432	56.65	<0.001
Present	9	54	63		
Total	285	210	495		
Corneal					
Absent	271	140	411	69.09	<0.001
Present	17	73	90		
Total	288	213	501		
Vestibular					
Absent	165	126	291	26.2	<0.001
Present	11	57	68		
Total	176	183	359		
Audio-ocular					
Absent	281	205	486	2.89	<0.1
Present	1	4	5		
Total	282	209	491		
Snout					
Absent	278	187	465	6.34	<0.02
Present	7	16	23		
Total	285	203	488		
Pharyngeal					
Absent	250	148	398	14.49	<0.001
Present	6	20	26		
Total	256	168	424		
Swallowing					
Absent	247	146	393	19.6	<0.001
Present	4	21	25		
Total	251	167	418		
Cough					
Absent	253	154	407	35.86	<0.001
Present	5	19	24		
Total	258	173	431		
Jaw Jerk					
Absent	272	168	440	17.96	<0.001
Present	10	29	39		
Total	282	197	479		

which did not have all the clinical manifestations of cerebral death, had low voltage slow activity on the scalp and from the depth electrodes rapid high voltage activity, the nature of which—biological or artifactual—was not clearly determined. However, it was concluded that electrocerebral silence on the scalp might well be associated with considerable activity in the depths.

This conclusion has been confirmed by others. Jonkman (220) reported the case of a 2-year-old child with encephalitis and absent scalp potentials. However, brainstem function was preserved, and depth electrodes showed subcortical electrical activity. Visser's (484) case was similar although apnea and ECS were present; depth electrodes recorded bursts of activity from the thalamus.

Evoked Potentials

The American EEG Society's Ad Hoc Committee on Cerebral Death (431) recommended that an attempt be made to evoke potentials by auditory, visual and tactile stimulation when recording on a patient suspected of cerebral death. Few reports on the findings have appeared, perhaps because the individual response is difficult to identify from the background activity without averaging techniques when biological activity is present, and when the tracing is flat a cortical potential is rarely evoked (51).

Trojaborg and Jorgensen (464) reported on the evoked responses in 50 comatose patients being artificially ventilated. In those cases with intact cranial nerve reflexes, visual and somatosensory cortical responses could be evoked, although the response was delayed and simple in form (without late components). In patients with no cephalic reflexes, induced somatosensory potentials and, rarely, visual potentials could be demonstrated. Auditory evoked potentials in patients with a dying brain have a long latency. As the brain dies, the potentials are of lower amplitude and with death lose their secondary components, so that eventually, if a response is obtained at all, it is only an attenuated wave I of long latency (448). Repetitive evoked electromyography in patients with a flat EEG produces a rapidly suppressed response that Kawai (237), who studied this phenomenon in 8 cases, concluded was a predictable sign of brain death. The conditioned negative shifts that may be induced by attention, expectancy, etc., in deeply comatose patients, require a greater number of paired stimuli to produce but do not differ morphologically from the responses in normal subjects (122).

Steady Potentials. The stationary potentials of the head are known to decrease with death. Manaka and Sano (299) found that in the normal human subject the steady potential, whether recorded from scalp or cortex, was approximately 20 mV above the potential of the nose. In cerebral death, this potential was reduced to zero, and in lesser degrees of brain hypoxia it decreased proportionally to the degree of brain damage. Bushart and Rittmeyer (80) also consider the DC negative shift to be a useful guide to cerebral death. They found that the usual response to hypoxia, a negative shift, was absent when cerebral circulation was abolished and the brain was dead.

Value of Electroencephalography in the Diagnosis of Cerebral Death

Since the early enthusiasm for the use of electroencephalography in determining a dead brain, considerable diversity of opinion has developed concerning its value. This has stemmed from a number of sources. Some neurologists have concluded that brain death can be made on clinical findings alone (104), others that EEG may be valuable as a confirmatory test (34), and still others consider it an essential examination for the diagnosis of a dead brain (155). Bennett (38) points out that the techniques for examining the brainstem reflexes are not well standardized and that even under research conditions as many as 10% may not be examined. If the diagnosis of brain death is made on a clinical basis, and one or two active cranial nerve reflexes are omitted from the examination, the spurious diagnosis of a dead brain may be made on the other criteria with no chance for an EEG to warn the observer of a possible remediable condition. It should be noted that 10% of cases meeting the clinical criteria of cerebral death according to certain authors (314, 327) will have biological activity in their electroencephalograms.

Hughes (199) points out that neither the presence nor the absence of biological activity is an indicator of a living or a dead brain. In a patient, comatose and even apneic due to a brainstem lesion, the EEG may have a good alpha rhythm (alpha coma). On the other hand, ECS may be present with all the clinical signs of brainstem life. Accordingly, brain death can only be assumed when all clinical and EEG criteria of a dead brain are met.

Comment.   An examination of the scalp potentials provides important and reliable information about brain activity in persons suspected of a dead brain. However, the resuscitative equipment, nursing services and labile cardiorespiratory state of the patient introduce artifactual material in these records. For this reason the interpretation of tracings requires more than average experience in reading EEGs. Provided the technical requirements of the American EEG Society for recording in cases of cerebral death are followed, ECS is reliable evidence of a nonfunctioning brain. To establish that the brain is dead solely on the basis of EEG findings requires multiple isoelectric recordings over 2 to 3 days. Although depth recordings or evoked potentials may give further evidence suggesting death, these techniques are too complicated for routine use. ECS in conjunction with a history of an irreparable lesion and clinical findings of an inactive brain is highly suggestive of a dead brain. However, if any aspects of the EEG are equivocal, or if the clinical data is incomplete, additional confirmatory tests are needed to substantiate the diagnosis of cerebral death.

Chapter VII

Neuropathological Findings in Cerebral Death

Introduction

It might be assumed that the pathological substrate of a dead brain would be a readily recognized morbid entity. Early, Bertrand et al. (46), impressed by the marked edema, softening and necrosis, especially pronounced in the gray matter, and the severe neuronal alterations without inflammatory reaction or vascular thrombosis, considered that these changes were characteristic of *coma dépassé*. Adams and Jequier (3) also described a fairly uniform pathological state in their 73 cases. However, Kramer (259), Lindenberg (289), Schneider et al. (413), and Walker et al. (498) have found more variable changes, the significance of which is not uniformly agreed upon. A review of the findings in the brains of patients whose cardiorespiratory system has been mechanically maintained illustrates the problem (498).

Gross Characteristics of the Brain and Spinal Cord

Weight. The encephalic weight is usually slightly above the normal range of brains matched for age and sex (Table VII–1). In the Collaborative

Table VII–1.   Relationship Between Brain Weight and Time on Respirator (192 Cases).

Hours on Respirator	Mean Weight of Brain at Autopsy (Kg)
0–11	1.43
12–23	1.45
24–47	1.38
48–71	1.44
72+	1.50

Study, those patients having resuscitative measures stopped on the basis of presumed cerebral death had heavier brains (by an average of 70 gms; $P = .014$) than those of patients succumbing to cardiac arrest. The sex distribution was similar in the two groups. Although the individuals having a cardiac death were, on the average, about 10 years older than those on whom resuscitation was stopped (48.6 vs. 36.1 years), among middle-aged people age-related differences in brain weight are minimal, so that the disparity is likely to be due to more congested and swollen brains in patients on whom resuscitation was stopped. The brains of persons dying within 24 hours from the beginning of resuscitative measures were heavier than those succumbing in the second day, but lighter than those of persons dying after 3 days.

Appearance.   The dura mater is usually well preserved and of normal color. The sagittal and/or transverse sinuses are clotted in 10–15% of cases; in most cases their walls appear normal. The spinal dura mater likewise seems normal, but the arachnoid may be distended by nodular fragments of cerebellar tissue in the subarachnoid or, less frequently, the subdural space.

On inspection, the encephalon of a person certified as cerebrally dead may be a well-preserved cerebrum or nondescript mushy mass. Some brains appear normal; others are soft, discolored and fragile, and a few so disintegrated that they cannot be removed from the calvarial cavity without fragmentation (Table VII–2). The swollen and congested cerebral hemispheres have a dusky hue. Transtentorial herniations are common. The brainstem is often torn and may be fragmented. The swollen cerebellum is molded about the edematous brainstem and cones into the foramen magnum, and sometimes the anterior lobe herniates into the incisura. The softened herniated cerebellar tonsils may be fragmented, with pieces of tonsillar tissue lodged along the spinal cord anywhere from the cervical segments to the cauda equina. Schneider and Matakas (412) have emphasized the occurrence of these cerebellar changes which they consider char-

Table VII–2. Relationship Between Condition of Brain and Time on Respirator.

		Hours on Respirator					
		0–11	12–23	24–27	48–71	72+	Total
Softening 217 Cases	Present	8 (53%)*	8 (42%)	44 (70%)	17 (55%)	62 (70%)	139 (64%)
Swelling 217 Cases	Present	12 (80%)	12 (63%)	49 (77%)	27 (87%)	62 (70%)	162 (75%)
Congestion 215 Cases	Present	8 (53%)	11 (61%)	40 (63%)	18 (58%)	53 (60%)	130 (60%)
Herniations 204 Cases	Present	8 (57%)	11 (65%)	48 (80%)	22 (73%)	48 (58%)	137 (67%)
Respirator brain 226 Cases	Present	2 (14%)	5 (26%)	32 (48%)	17 (51%)	35 (38%)	91 (40%)

*The percentages are the ratio of cases having the pathological condition to the number of cases in the time class.

acteristic of brain death when it has been present more than 36 hours. In addition, hemorrhagic softening of the upper few segments of the cervical spinal cord occurs but often is overlooked, misinterpreted or that part of the central nervous system is not removed or inspected. Even though the brain is placed in a fixative soon after its removal, the tissues may not harden but remain gelatinous (Figure VII–1).

In about 10% of cases, the cut sections appear grossly normal, but in more than half of the brains the white matter is edematous and soft. Numerous petechial hemorrhages are present in the cortex and to a lesser extent in the subcortical ganglia. The primary lesion may be responsible for additional local or diffuse changes as well as herniations through the tentorial notch or foramen magnum. The cut surface of the cerebellum appears wet, and the folia are less well demarcated from the adjacent white matter than usual. The brainstem, if not distorted by hemorrhages, is soft, friable and may be lacerated (Figure VII–2).

Sections of the cervicomedullary junction and upper segments of the spinal cord often have superficial areas of necrosis and hemorrhage where tonsillar herniations compressed the cord. Because, rostrally, the vertebral artery supplying the medulla is usually occluded, and, caudally, the blood supply from the spinal arteries remains intact, a zone of edema, laceration, and petechial hemorrhages demarcates the spinomedullary junction. In some cases, perivascular infiltrations in the lower cervical segments of the spinal cord are evidence of an intact circulation. Unfortunately, this part of the cervical cord is often not examined at autopsy, so that the true incidence of these pathological changes at the cervicomedullary junction is not known.

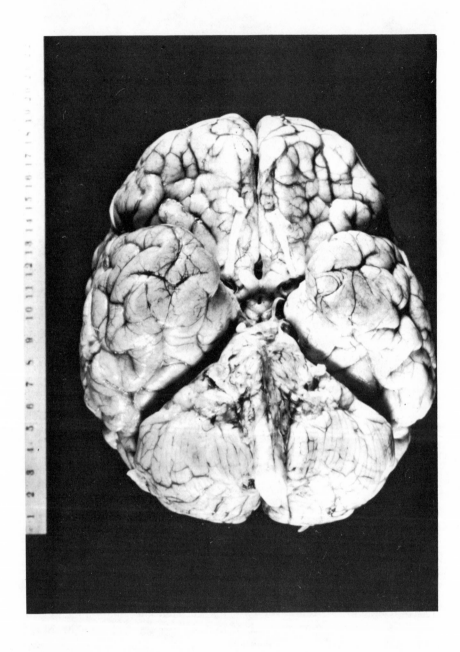

Fig. VII–1. Basal surface of the brain from a patient who had been artificially ventilated. Note the swollen convolutions with narrowed sulci, the tonsillar coning and molding about the medulla oblongata.

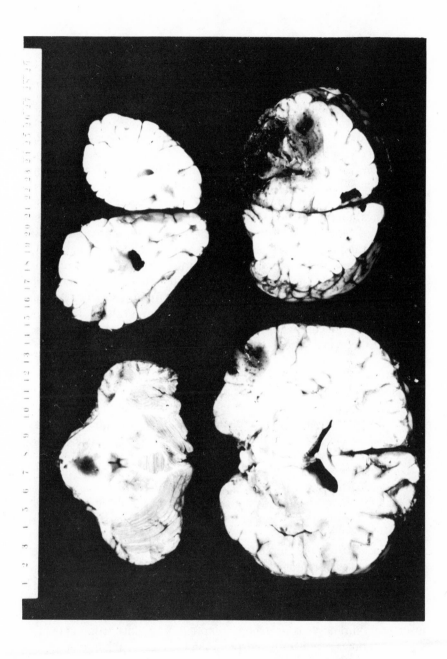

Fig. VII–2. Sections of a traumatized brain from a patient artificially ventilated for 24 hours. Hemorrhagic infiltrations and edema of the right frontal lobe, patchy necrosis in the cerebellar folia and central pontine hemorrhages are apparent.

Histopathological Alterations

Microscopically, the brains and spinal cords of brain-death cases vary from essentially a normal to a severely disintegrated nervous system.

Spinal Cord.   The spinal cord usually appears normal, but in perhaps a third of the cases edema, neurolysis, hemorrhage and, rarely, infarction of segments are noted. The myelinated tracts of the cord appear normal. In some cases, a spectacular migration and lodgment of cerebellar fragments in the spinal subarachnoid space may be seen grossly as nodular thickenings, and in stained sections as bits of cerebellar folia. These variously sized blobs of necrotic and fairly well preserved cerebellar tissue are lodged about the nerve roots at any level in the subarachnoid or, less commonly, the subdural space. Usually little or no inflammatory reaction is seen at the site of these folial deposits, although Schneider and Matakas (412) have described a foreign body reaction to fragments when the patient has been on the respirator for several days (Figure VII–3). This response to the presence of cerebellar fragments might be expected since the vascular supply to the spinal cord is still intact.

Brainstem.   The brainstem appears normal in about 15% of the cases, but commonly edema, hemorrhage, infarction, necrosis and/or neuronal loss occur. Since the lower medulla oblongata bears the brunt of the displacement and herniation of the cerebellar tonsils, it is frequently flattened. The pons is usually edematous, necrotic and hemorrhagic, especially about its periphery.

   The mesencephalon is distorted by local edema or external compression by herniating tissue of the medial temporal structures or the anterior cerebellar lobes. As a result, ischemic or hemorrhagic softenings and flame-shaped or confluent midline or peri-aqueductal hemorrhages are often present (Figure VII–4).

   The location of the herniation predicates its effect upon the mesencephalon and surrounding structures. An anterior transtentorial herniation may displace the pituitary stalk, resulting in thromboses and other vascular lesions of the hypophysis. In lateral transtentorial herniations, hippocampal cortex is compressed by the sharp edge of the tentorium and the ipsilateral third nerve is stretched; compression and distortion of the brainstem sometimes produces hemorrhages in the mesencephalon or about the aqueduct of Sylvius. The herniation may occlude the posterior cerebral artery as it passes over the sharp edge of the tentorium to reach the supratentorial cavity and the calcarine cortex. A more posterior or midline herniation depresses and flattens the quadrigeminal plate and the cerebral

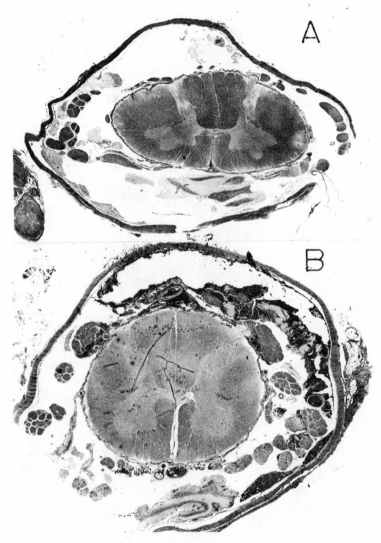

Fig. VII–3. Sections of the cervical (A) and thoracic (B) spinal cords to show the deposits of macerated cerebellar folia in the subarachnoid spaces with no inflammatory reaction. (Hematoxylin and eosin, (H&E; A, X6, and B, X8)

peduncles. With a herniation in this location, there is likely to be displacement and tension upon the perforating vessels from the posterior cerebral arteries to the cerebral peduncle and to the pons from the basilar artery, causing brainstem hemorrhages.

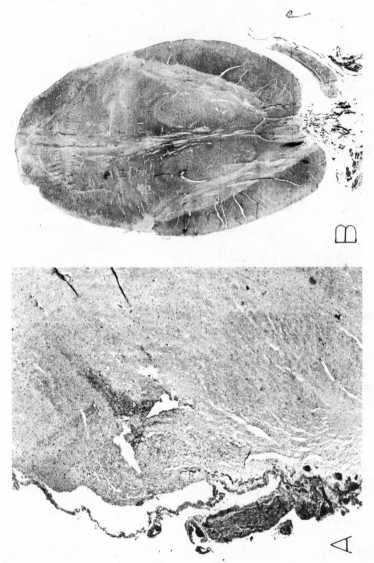

Fig. VII–4. A and B. Sections from the Brainstem.

A   Macerated spinomedullary junction with edema and small hemorrhagic infiltrates (H&E: X25).
B   Distorted compressed mesencephalon with edema and a few hemorrhages in the interpeduncular region (H&E: X4).

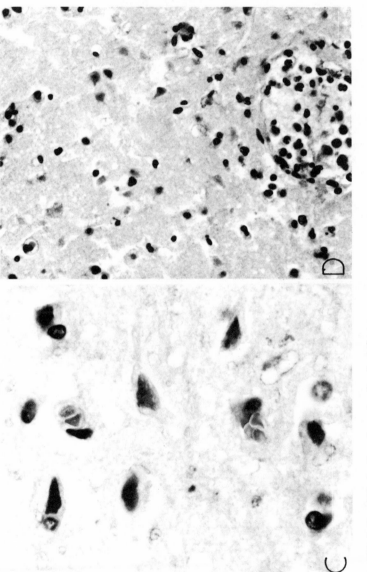

Fig. VII-4, C and D. Sections from the Cerebral Cortex.

C   Cortical neurons with pyknotic nuclei, vacuolated homogenous cytoplasm and pericellular edema (H&E; X1000).

D   Cortical softening with engorged capillary, edematous tissue, shrunken neurons with pyknotic nuclei and homogenous pale cytoplasm, gitter and small round cells (H&E; X500).

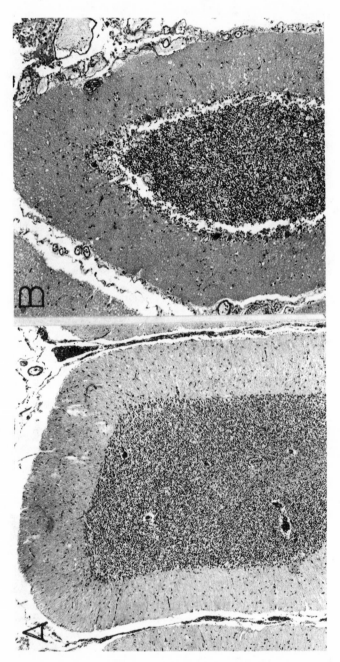

Fig. VII-5, A and B. Sections from the Cerebellum.

A   Severe lysis of a cerebellar folium with absence of most of the granular and Purkinje cells. The molecular layer is better preserved (H&E; X50).

B   Marked edema of the Purkinje cell layer with only a few pyknotic cells remaining (H&E; X70).

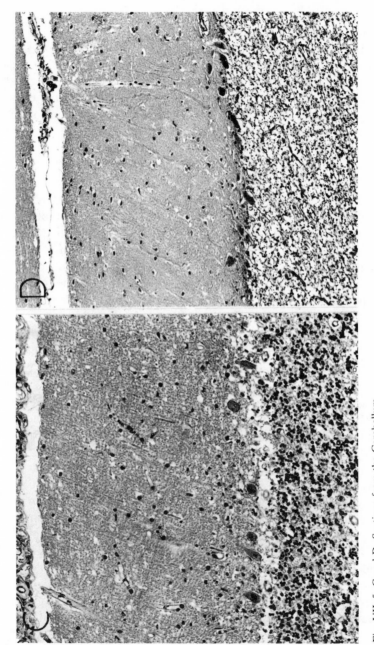

Fig. VII–5, C and D. Sections from the Cerebellum.

C   Moderate lysis of granular cells, edema and anoxic changes of the Purkinje cells (H&E; X175).

D   Severe lysis of granular cells and pyknotic Purkinje cells (H&E; X125).

Cerebellum.   Although 10% of cerebella appear normal, the posterior fossa structures are severely compromised in most cases of cerebral death. The striking feature on microscopic examination is the swelling and congestion of the cerebellar hemispheres. In more than half of the cases, the cerebellar folia, normally densely stained by aniline dyes, have a washed out appearance due to the failure of the granular layer to take the dye. The degree of the lytic process varies from case to case and may not correspond to the amount of damage to the Purkinje cell layer, which may be almost normal or edematous and/or completely devoid of cells. The molecular layer is usually well preserved (Figure VII–5).

Diencephalon.   The diencephalon, often devoid of frank hemorrhages or softenings, is usually said to be relatively spared in the brain of the cerebrally dead. However, some degree of neuronal damage is present in almost 85% of cases. The most common histological lesion of the periventricular regions is edema, but patchy lytic changes are frequently seen in the neurons. Small hypothalamic infarcts or softenings due to displacement and compression by transtentorial herniations may be present.

Cortex.   The cerebral cortex is the most frequently and severely damaged part of the brain. Rarely is there no cortical lesion. The pathological alterations in the cerebral hemispheres in some cases are due to occlusion of vascular channels. Frank infarcts of the occipital, temporal or frontal lobes result from occlusion of posterior, middle or anterior cerebral arteries respectively. The infarcts are usually hemorrhagic and involve the cortex more than the adjacent white matter. The occlusion may be a thrombosis of a major vessel due to intrinsic vascular disease such as atherosclerosis, or it may be the result of compression of an artery against a rigid structure such as the tentorium. More commonly, however, the cerebral cortex is diffusely congested and edematous, and the cortical neurones exhibit various degrees of acute ischemic change, characterized by dark staining nuclei and, in hemotoxylin and eosin preparations, a pink staining cytoplasm. In spite of the marked edema and regressive neuronal alterations, there is no evidence of glial or hematogenous reaction.

If the patient survives for days, islands of neurons with chronic ischemic changes in lytic zones are scattered throughout the cortex. In places, these chronic changes take the form of a laminar necrosis. In general, the cerebral cortex is more severely involved than the white matter. Only in the brains of patients surviving long periods of time are multiple and diffuse lesions of the white matter associated with preserved areas of the cortex.

Pituitary. Patients with cerebral death have from mild to severe changes in the pituitary gland. Grossly, the gland may appear normal, be brown or softened. Petechiae are present in about half of these glands.

McCormick and Halmi (313) have described the histological changes in these pituitaries. In the pars nervosa, small petechia to confluent hemorrhages were present in 12 of 24 cases in their series; necrosis was seen in 10 cases. In the pars distalis, pyknosis of the eosinophil cells and foci of detached cells were constant features; however, in 88% of cases, severe degenerative changes with detachment of cells from the basement membrane, with or without areas of necrosis and softening, were present. These changes, particularly the fresh infarcts, were much more frequently found in patients who had been on a respirator than in general autopsy material. Karyopyknotic and desquamative changes of the anterior pituitary lobe are the most characteristic pituitary alterations in patients who die in *coma dépassé*.

Comment. These pathological changes in the brains of comatose persons maintained on a respirator have emphasized the severe autolytic alterations in the cerebral and cerebellar cortices without evidence of reactive changes (154, 245, 258, 411). Fuchs and Schneider (139) showed that in the first hour after arrest of CBF, the vasculature of the brain was little damaged so that if the blood flow was restored, a normal circulation ensued. However, longer ischaemic periods produced changes in the vessel walls, so that with the resumption of blood flow hemorrhages occurred in the basal ganglia and cortex. In addition a polymorphonuclear reaction was seen about cortical vessels.

Respirator Brain

The above described constellation of pathological changes found in the brains of people following periods of artificial respiration have been termed the "respirator brain." In brief, the respirator brain, according to Kimura et al. (245) and the majority of American neuropathologists (337), consists of edema and softening of the entire brain, grayish-brown discoloration of gray matter, nonadherent clots in the dural sinuses, pale swollen cerebellar folia and often necrotic and sloughing tonsillar herniations. Microscopic changes include diffuse anoxic necrosis of cerebral cortical neurons, marked autolysis of the cerebellar structures, particularly pronounced in the granular cell layer, and generally, pallor of myelin. These changes are characteristic of brains of patients who have been on artificial respiration.

These alterations are essentially the same as Kramer (258) described as intravital brain death and considered to be typical of "deanimation," his term for cerebral death (Table VII–3). Schneider et al. (411) believe that neither the gross nor histological findings in the brains of individuals maintained for a short time on a respirator—swelling of the brain, structural disintegration, and profuse congestion of veins and arteries—are pathognomonic of brain death. They aver that only after 36 hours of brain death do the more specific changes appear—namely, herniation and fragmentation of necrotic cerebellar tissue into the spinal subarachnoid space, hemorrhagic softening of the upper cervical segments, and necrosis of the anterior lobe of the pituitary gland. Thus, Schneider et al. (411) consider that there are nonspecific as well as specific changes in the brains of persons suffering cerebral death. However, they admit that these changes cannot be demonstrated, even when sought for, if the period between death of the brain and of the organism is short—in other words, if the period of artificial ventilation is brief. Moreover, the morphologic picture may be incomplete, i.e., not all of the findings may be present.

Some neuropathologists point out that certain of these changes are almost indistinguishable from the postmortem alterations resulting from delayed fixation, or from storage of the cadaver at temperatures over 35° C. Some features—swelling and discoloration of the brain, and ischemic neurons—are particularly prominent in respirator brains, while softening and necrosis are more common in postmortem autolysis. Even the more experienced neuropathologists have difficulty in differentiating the changes when both anoxic and autolytic factors operate to varying degrees in different parts of the brain. For these reasons some neuropathologists do not credit the concept of respirator brain as a specific entity, but believe that the changes are simply the result of postmortem autolysis. Lindenberg (289) has answered this charge more precisely than most neuropathologists. He points out that premortal cerebral processes such as ischemia may continue to operate after cardiac arrest and utilize enzyme systems which otherwise would participate in the autolytic phenomenon. Consequently, after a chronic illness, the cerebral neurons may seem better preserved than when death occurs suddenly. Steegmann's observation (449) that severe cell changes may be associated with a 5-minute cardiac arrest would confirm this thesis.

But this hypothesis does not appeal to many neuropathologists, especially the Europeans, who share the view "that the changes in the 'respirator brain' are autolytic phenomena, and that there can therefore be no vital reaction on the part of tissues; thus neurons and parenchyma show

Table VII–3.   Neuropathological Changes in Brains of Comatose and Apneic Persons
(modified from Kramer).

	Grade 1 (slight)	Grade 2 (moderate)	Grade 3 (severe)
Macroscopic			
Consistency	Soft	Softer	Semi-liquid
Localization	Circumscribed	Extensive	Entire brain
Color	Yellow	Yellow-brown	Yellow-green
Microscopic			
Staining quality	Poor	Very poor	Minimal
Ground sub-			
stance	Darkly stained	Darkly stained	Palely stained
Edema	Perivascular	Generalized	Peri- and intracellular
Vessels	Engorged	R.B.C.'s lysed	Necrotic capillary wall with R.B.C. diapedesis. Tissue continuity destroyed
Neurons	Swollen	Swollen	Loss of cell structure
Cytoplasm	Meta- and hyperchromatic Loss of Nissl bodies	Metachromatic homogeneous. pale or darkly stained, vacuolated and granular	Liquefaction and vacuolization
Nucleus	Eccentric	Pyknotic or pale and vacuolated	Pyknotic and fragmented
Glia	Swollen Metachromatic Clasmatodendrosis	Swollen, vacuolated with pyknotic nucleus	Liquefied and foamy
White matter	Myelin preserved	Swollen, fragmented myelin sheaths	Edematous, swollen myelin. Irregular axons

cytolysis and autolysis rather than ischemic change and necrosis. For this reason also inflammatory changes and gliosis cannot occur in the 'respirator brain.' Conventional reactive changes and classical alterations in neurons may of course precede the onset of 'respirator brain change,' and may still be recognizable if autolysis is not too advanced. The combination of neuronal loss and gliomesodermal reactions that are related to survival time from a particular incident is very different from the process of autolysis, and the two should be distinguishable" (2).

Obviously, it is impossible at the present time to arrive at a unanimous interpretation of these findings. However, in order to examine the relationship of this constellation of findings to other phenomena associated with cerebral death, they will be collectively considered as a pathological entity called the respirator brain in the following discussion.

Factors in the Development of a Respirator Brain

If one considers a respirator brain as simply an autolysed cerebrum, its development should have little relationship to antecedent conditions. However, if the respirator brain is dependent upon vital enzyme systems and metabolic stores, the state of the brain preceding and following its death may well predicate its later metamorphosis. An examination of some of the possible contributing factors may help to clarify the issues.

Time on the Respirator.   That the duration of mechanical aeration plays a role in the pathogenesis of a respirator brain has been discussed by a number of neuropathologists without their arriving at a unanimous opinion. Although some investigators (289) have suggested a causal relationship, the clearest evidence has come from the Collaborative Study (Table VII–4). Of the patients artificially ventilated up to 12 hours, only two had brains classified as respirator brains; of 19 patients on the respirator for 12 to 23.9 hours, 5 had respirator brains; and of 67 patients artificially aerated for 24 to 47.9 hours, 32 were considered to have respirator brains. Approximately half (36 of 74) of the patients on the respirator for 48 to 144 hours had brains classified as respirator brains, and thereafter the percentage dropped to approximately 33%. This sequence suggests that a period of time, approximately 24 hours, is required for the changes characterizing a respirator brain to develop.

This 24-hour time period is within the range stated by a number of pathologists. In 1963, Greenfield and Meyer (160) concluded that 14–15 hours survival after an anoxic episode was necessary for neuronal changes to be demonstrated by light microscopy.

Table VII–4.   Relationship of Time on Respirator to Respirator Brain.

Time on Respirator (Hours)	Number of Cases	Respirator Brain	
		No	Yes
<12	15	13	2 (13%)
12–23.9	19	14	5 (26%)
24–47.9	67	35	32 (48%)
48–71.9	33	16	17 (51%)
72–95.9	25	15	10 (40%)
96–119.9	16	7	9 (56%)
120–143.9	12	7	5 (42%)
144–167.9	6	4	2 (33%)
>168	33	24	9 (27%)

Nedey et al. (343), on the basis of the examination of 18 cases of cerebral death, concluded that unless the subject had been on the respirator at least 24 hours the changes in the brain were minimal. This is also very close to the conclusions of Schneider et al. (411), who considered that 36 hours would have to elapse before the findings became specific. However, other writers have denied a relationship between time on respirator and respirator brain (248).

Relationship of Primary Diagnosis to Neuropathological Findings

It has been claimed that the state of the brain before a lethal ictus determines the type of necrobiosis which ensues. If so, it should play an important role in the development of a respirator brain. The major clinical conditions causing brain death are listed in Table VII–5 with the percentage of respirator brains in each group. With the exception of cerebral trauma and intoxications, it would seem that the percentage of respirator brains in each category is quite similar. In head injury, the high percentage of respirator brains (52% as compared with an average of 40% for the other categories) may be related to the great number of cases with acute intracranial hypertension. In the exo- and endogenous intoxications, the low proportion of respirator to nonrespirator brains (25%) may be attributed

Table VII–5.   Relationship of Primary Diagnosis to Respirator Brain.

Primary Diagnosis	Type of Brain (Percentage)		
	Non-respirator	Respirator	Total
All	135 (60%)	91 (40%)	226
Cardiac	27 (64%)	15 (36%)	42
Trauma	25 (48%)	27 (52%)	52
Cerebrovascular:			
Thrombosis	6 (46%)	7 (54%)	13
S A H......................	11 (55%)	9 (45%)	20
Embolism	4 —	— —	4
Hemorrhage	14 (53%)	12 (47%)	26
Other	5 —	1 —	6
Total Cerebrovascular	40 (56%)	29 (44%)	69
Infection	7 (64%)	4 (36%)	11
Exogenous Intoxication	4 —	— —	4
Metabolic	15 (71%)	6 (29%)	21
Neoplasm	3 —	2 —	5
Other	14 (64%)	8 (36%)	22

to the depressant effects of intoxicants on anaerobic glycolysis; the observation is in line with the experimental finding that barbiturates lessen the extent of anoxic infarction (337).

Relationship of Vital Signs to Neuropathological Findings

Failure of vital functions—temperature, pulse rate and blood pressure—although indicative of brainstem involvement, do not seem to be responsible for specific neuropathological lesions. In patients with respirator brains, there is a tendency for the temperatures to be subnormal (Table VII–6); a comparison of the percent of respirator brains obtained from patients with a final temperature below 95° with those taken from patients with terminal fevers above 100° F indicated a significantly smaller ratio (P = 0.01). The systolic blood pressure relates weakly to occurrence of respirator brains. When the systolic blood pressure is below 70 mm Hg, the ratio of respirator to non-respirator brains is increased (Table VII–7).

Relationship of Cephalic Reflexes to Neuropathological Findings

The cephalic reflexes are quite sensitive to anoxic stress. Table VII–8 indicates some variation in the number of cephalic reflexes that were absent at the time of the final examination in a series of comatose and apneic patients. The low rates for pharyngeal and swallowing reflexes might be

Table VII–6.   Relationship of Rectal Temperature to Respirator Brain.

| Temperature (°F) | Respirator Brain | | | | | |
| | No | | Yes | | Totals | |
	Initial	Final	Initial	Final	Initial	Final
0–90	2	6	6	4	8	10
91–95	14	25	11	21	25	46
96–100	74	61	44	51	118	112
101–105	43	40	30	15	73	55
106+	2	3	—	—	2	3
Totals	135	135	91	91	226	226

Table VII–7.   Relationship of systolic Blood Pressure to Respirator Brain.

| Systolic B.P. (mm Hg) | Respirator Brain | | | | | |
| | No | | Yes | | Total | |
	Initial	Final	Initial	Final	Initial	Final
0–50	12	19	11	18	23	37
51–70	8	11	12	13	20	24
71–90	19	29	14	19	33	48
91–110	38	34	23	20	61	54
111–130	19	21	15	14	34	35
131–150	17	13	8	2	25	15
151–170	11	5	3	4	14	9
171 + ...	11	3	5	1	16	4
Totals	135	135	91	91	226	226

Table VII–8.   Relationship of Cephalic Reflexes (Final Examination) to Respirator Brain.

| Reflex Present | Respirator Brain | |
	No (135 cases)	Yes (91 cases)
Pupillary reaction to light	22%	5%
Corneal reflex	18%	3%
Oculocephalic reflex	14%	4%
Vestibular	13%	4%
Swallowing	7%	1%
Snout	7%	3%
Pharyngeal	4%	1%
Audio-ocular	3%	—

attributed to local conditions in the throat, such as intratracheal or nasogastric tubes or local dehydration.

However, a much smaller proportion of persons with respirator brains had small pupils (27%) than large pupils (50%). Along the same line, persons with pupils reactive to light were unlikely to have respirator brains; only 5% of respirator brain cases had a pupillary reflex. The corneal reflexes were absent in almost 90% of cases and in about 97% of cases in which the total picture of the respirator brain was present. A high percentage of the other cephalic reflexes were absent when the gross appearance was compatible with that of a respirator brain.

In general, a decrease in cephalic reflex activity is associated with an increase in number of respirator brains and vice versa.

Relationship of Spinal Reflexes to Neuropathological Findings

The presence of the spinal reflexes, both superficial and deep, does not correlate well with the presence or absence of a respirator brain. As might be expected, the respirator brain is more common when the reflexes are in abeyance. The presence (22% of cases) and location of histological changes in the spinal cord do not correlate with the state of the reflexes.

Relationship of Medication to Neuropathological Findings

In view of the known sedative and anti-inflammatory effects of certain medications, one might expect to find evidence of their action in the autopsy material. However, the presence of barbiturates in the blood in about half of the autopsied cases had no apparent influence upon the neuropathological picture nor upon the likelihood of a respirator brain. Swelling of the brain was just as frequent in the patients receiving analgesics (45%) as in those receiving antibiotic agents (42%) or corticosteroids (45%). Nor were there significant differences in the number of brains with congestion, discoloration or herniations that might be related to the ingestion of different classes of drugs.

This incidence of respirator brains might have been influenced by medications, since such drugs as corticosteroids theoretically should decrease anoxic lesions. However, cases treated with antibiotics had 37% respirator brains, with vasopressors 33%, and with corticosteroids 45%; the mean of the entire series was 40%.

Relationship of Therapy to Neuropathological Findings

Such therapies as hypothermia, dialysis, etc., might be considered to produce some effect upon the pathological condition of the brain, but its appearance did not seem to be changed by any of these therapies.

Relationship of EEG to Neuropathological Findings

A priori, one would assume that a dead brain should be associated with an isoelectric record of the brain waves. As seen in Table VII–9, cases with biological activity in the last EEG recorded are associated with few swollen brains, fewer cerebral herniations and fewer respirator brains than cases without evidence of electrical activity in the electroencephalograms. The patients with EEGs diagnosed as equivocal seem to comprise a group with pathological changes between the other two classes.

A flat EEG is more likely to be associated with a pathological diagnosis of hemorrhage than infarction; other conditions have a relatively low percentage of isoelectric records (Table VII–10).

The location of the pathology bears a relationship to the probability of electrocerebral silence, for patients with diffuse or focal cerebral lesions are much more likely to have ECS than persons with other lesions.

The state of the brain waves also relates to the likelihood of a respirator brain. Although ECS is present in many cases that do not have a respirator brain, an active EEG correlates highly with a nonrespirator brain (Table VII–9). There is a trend for more respirator brains to occur in cases with hemorrhage, edema, and necrosis, but a normal spinal cord is compatible with an average number of respirator brains (Table VII–10).

It is logical to expect that there should be a high correlation of respirator brain with those clinical manifestations suggesting a functionless brain. In general, this is the case, but there are a few exceptions. Some of these may be dismissed summarily on the basis that the brain wave records were made days before death, so that there is the possibility that an immediate premortem EEG would have demonstrated ECS. But, irrespective of defections, the presence of muscle fasciculations, electrocardiographic tracings, movement and other adventitious pen deflections simulating an active EEG, the final records of some persons with brains diagnosed as respirator have had biological activity unobscured by artifact. The pathological findings in these cases were atypical because of patchy swelling, edema, infarction and necrosis.

Relationship of Cerebral Circulation to Neuropathological Findings

It has been asserted that cerebral death is the result of a total brain infarction. A careful neuropathological study of brains in which the CBF

Table VII-9.   Relationship of Appearance of Brain to Last EEG.

| | | Appearance of Brain (Percentage) | | | | | | | |
| | | Swelling | | | Herniations | | | Respirator Brain | |
EEG	Number	None	Generalized	Other	None	Transtentorial	Other	No	Yes
Equivocal	14	2 (14%)	8 (57%)	4 (29%)	3 (21%)	10 (71%)	1 (7%)	10 (71%)	4 (29%)
Biological activity	67	36 (54%)	13 (19%)	18 (27%)	42 (63%)	15 (22%)	10 (15%)	58 (87%)	9 (13%)
Electrocerebral silence	144	16 (11%)	91 (63%)	37 (26%)	21 (15%)	93 (65%)	30 (21%)	66 (46%)	78 (54%)

Table VII-10.   Relationship of Type and Location of Lesion to Last EEG.

| | Total Number of Cases (Percentage with Biological Activity*) | | | | | |
| | | Location of Lesion | | | | |
Type of Lesion	Cortex	Diencephalon	Cerebellum	Brainstem	Medulla	Spinal Cord
None	11 (55%)	38 (42%)	36 (50%)	35 (49%)	96 (38%)	76 (38%)
Infarction	38 (39%)	28 (43%)	23 (48%)	27 (40%)	7 (14%)	3 (0%)
Hemorrhage	32 (9%)	28 (4%)	18 (11%)	36 (22%)	4 (0%)	5 (20%)
Edema	63 (22%)	46 (13%)	37 (14%)	42 (5%)	27 (0%)	16 (13%)
Necrosis or lysis	26 (42%)	24 (46%)	42 (19%)	23 (21%)	13 (15%)	6 (0%)
Neuronal loss	29 (45%)	29 (52%)	32 (44%)	23 (61%)	8 (22%)	8 (38%)
Other	12 (42%)	19 (29%)	23 (36%)	25 (38%)	58 (63%)	102 (31%)

*Remainder of cases had ECS (cases with equivocal EEGs eliminated)

was absent and brains in which CBF was to some extent intact has been reported by Pearson et al. (369). In six brains from patients with absent bolus studies at least 20 hours before cardiac arrest, the typical findings of a respirator brain were present. The authors considered the changes as autolysis such as could be seen when brains have been kept warm after death. On the other hand, six brains from patients who had a head bolus at least 20 hours before cardiac arrest showed focal necrosis with intact but swollen vascular endothelium. Phagocytic cells were present in the necrotic areas and astrocytes showed reactive changes. The cerebellum and brainstem were generally undamaged.

This differential neuropathological finding seems to confirm the hypothesis that the dead brain is due to a cerebral vascular arrest. However, a number of questions remain unanswered. What happens to the focal necrotic areas of the brain when CBF arrests more than 24 hours after the primary insult? Can the reactive changes in these brains be identified after the later infarction? Perhaps the varied neuropathological picture in cerebral death cases may be explicable on such a basis.

Discussion

In spite of the difficulties in classifying the variegated pathology in the brains of patients dying after protracted coma, the set of neuropathological findings characterizing the respirator brain syndrome has positive correlations with certain clinical and electroencephalographic findings. It would seem that the development of a respirator brain is a dynamic process that may go on after pulmonary and/or cardiac arrest, or after resuscitation has been stopped; to what degree the changes in the central nervous system represent a stage of acute cerebral ischemia or cerebral acidosis is difficult to determine in any one case, just as it is impossible to assess the role of autolytic necrobiosis. In many brains both factors may have been operative.

A number of neuropathologists have noted the varying changes in the brains of people who have been in deep irreversible coma. Kramer (258) has described these changes in cases of deanimation. Lindenberg (289) attempted to explain the differences on the basis of the premorbid state of the central nervous system. He believed that if the brain was hypoxic prior to an acute arrest of circulation, the encephalic structures would develop few changes (morphostatic necrobiosis); whereas if there was no such protective event, the brain rapidly underwent necrotic changes (morphotrophic necrobiosis). Perhaps this is in line with the observations of Myers and Yamaguchi (341) that food-deprived monkeys may recover from 10-minute arrest of cerebral circulation, whereas glucose-infused animals develop myoclonic seizures and die within 2 days. The brains of the food-deprived animals show no significant injury, whereas the brains of the fed animals are edematous, swollen and have an impaired blood-brain barrier. Moreover, varied biochemical changes occur after circulatory arrest. In food-deprived animals, ATP is decreased to 0.08 μmoles/g, lactate is moderately increased to 12.08 μmoles/g, and NaK-activated ATPase activity is increased. After a similar period of arrest in fed animals, the ATP is 0.14 μmoles/g and lactate is 32.5 μmoles/g.

Lindenberg (289) believes that an intra- and pericellular acidosis develops at the rate of 0.15 of 1 pH/min. This creates an optimal environment for the activity of hydrolytic enzymes contained within lysosomes that swell and break down, causing a disturbance in osmotic balance. This dysosmosis induces a marked uptake of water by cells and interstitial tissues. Within six hours, the acidotic dysosmosis produces severe edema of the gray and white matter. The vascular endothelium swells and takes up watery vacuoles. This endothelial swelling reduces the size of the lumen, which then becomes plugged with deformed erythrocytes, Matakas et al. (310) emphasize that within 12 to 48 hours the capillary lumen is obstructed by endothelial swelling, erythrocytes or blebs. However, Lindenberg implies that if the circulation is intact considerable amounts of lactic acid may be discharged into and carried away by the blood stream, thus preventing an acidotic dysosmosis. He contends that a chronic hypoxemia before acute ischemia will lower the phosphocreatinine, ATP and ADP content, so that what little glucose is present cannot be metabolized, even in the anaerobic cycle, and so lactic acid is kept at nontoxic levels. A preliminary hypoxemia of 20 minutes, according to Lindenberg, is sufficient to produce a morphostatic rather than a morphotrophic necrobiosis.

Most European authors now define brain death as the survival of the organism after the complete and permanent arrest of cerebral circulation, and believe that the most reliable sign of cerebral death is the demonstration of the absence of cerebral circulation by angiography. Basically, two factors have been shown to be important in the development of these pathological changes within the brain. The first is the critical perfusion pressure, defined as the difference between the mean systemic arterial blood pressure and the cerebral venous pressure. The second is the critical oxygen tension. The relationship between the critical profusion pressure and the critical oxygen tension is important, for an imbalance leads to the accumulation of toxic products of metabolic degradation, such as lactic acid.

The roles of these two factors may be tested by analyzing two types of cerebral death. Akin to the common technique for inducing experimental cerebral ischemia—the inflation of a balloon or some other space-occupying device in the subdural or extradural space—are the traumatic and vascular lesions which increase the intracranial pressure above the systolic blood pressure, producing an arrest of CBF and a rapid and severe cerebral ischemia. The other cerebral death syndrome is produced by cardiac arrest, in which there is a failure of adequate profusion of the intracranial contents, but not necessarily an immediate ischemia of the brain.

If the above theory is true, the pathological alterations following these two types of brain death should differ. To test this, the neuropathological findings in patients with cerebral trauma and with primary heart disease have been compared. The first group of cases suffer from a critical loss of oxygen and the second from impaired critical profusion pressure. In Table VII–11, a number of factors have been analyzed. It is apparent that the EEG findings differ significantly in the two groups (P = 0.000001), for many more patients have biological activity in the first group than in the second. In traumatic cases, there are many more brains with cerebral herniations than in cardiac cases (P = 0.0003). Thus, it seems that cardiac disease associated with impaired profusion pressure tends to result in cerebral infarctions and severe ischemic changes, and the traumatic cases with decreased oxygen tension produce cerebral herniations and hemorrhages.

Table VII–11.   Comparison of EEG and Neuropathological Factors in Cases of Cardiac Disease and Cerebral Trauma (Final Examination).

Electroencephalogram	Cardiac Disease	Cerebral Trauma
Biological Activity	62 (5)*	15 (7)*
Electrocerebral Silence	36	72
Time (ECS to death)		
0–5.9 hours	9	13
6–11.9	4	6
12–23.9	8	18
24–47.9	11	25
48–71.9	3	4
72–95.9	1	1
96	—	5
Herniation		
None	20	6
Present	27	48
Neuropathological Diagnosis		
Normal	2	—
Infarction	14	3
Hemorrhage	5	29
Trauma	3	19
Tumor	1	—
Edema	9	—
Other or Unknown	13	3
Respirator Brain		
None	27	25
Present	15	27

*Equivocal records

These findings confirm the hypothesis that the brains of individuals with cerebral death due to different pathogenetic factors do differ pathologically, at least in some respects.

Summary

Although there are many gradations in the pathological findings in the brains of persons who have been sustained on a respirator, there emerges from the findings a morbid entity that most neuropathologists consider a respirator brain. The pathogenesis of this state is not entirely clear. It is more commonly found when cerebral trauma, hemorrhage or thrombosis is the primary or causative lesion, and is less frequently present in primary vascular (cardiac) and metabolic states. Perhaps the causative mechanism in these cases relates more to physical (intracranial pressure) attributes than to the biological aspects of the primary lesion, but this has not been conclusively demonstrated. Such secondary factors as treatment (physical or pharmacological) age or hormonal disturbances do not seem to play significant roles. Even posthypoxic edema per se, according to Nicholson et al. (350), is not sufficient to account for the lesions.

More evidence is accumulating to indicate that intra- and extracellular acidosis plays a major role in the process of brain death. The severe acidosis from lactic acid, generated by anaerobic cellular metabolism, deranges membranes and cellular enzymes, so that edema of neurons, glia and interstitial tissue results. If this acidosis can be lessened by being washed out by a certain amount of cerebral blood flow (194) or by depletion of metabolites before the anoxic insult (319), the pathological changes may be averted or minimized. However, in most cases of respirator dependency, the period of mechanical ventilation is sufficiently long that autolytic changes occur in the incubated brain. The precise chemical nature of these alterations is poorly understood, but unquestionably they must be related to the tissue metabolism and enzymes. Moreover, they are operative over periods of time which may be as long as several days. It would seem likely that at their inception these autolytic changes are dependent upon the biochemical state of the brain. This transition would seem to be inherent to the concept of morphotrophic and morphostatic necrosis (288). Hence, although Kramer (260) divides the clinical and pathological course into stages, there is no sharp divison either clinically or pathologically. The fact that a pathological end point can not be attained until long after the brain has ceased functioning (if at all) makes a definition of the moment of death on clinical or instrumental findings both arbitrary and theoretical.

Chapter VIII

Criteria of Cerebral Death

Introduction

Only in the middle of the twentieth century, when physicians turned their attention to developing techniques that would provide basic life support for comatose individuals, was consideration given to the possibility of introducing a new method to determine death. The use of external cardiac massage to stimulate an asystolic heart and of artificial respirators to provide gaseous exchange were often successful in restoring cardiac activity, but, at times, only after the circulation had been arrested so long that the organ most sensitive to oxygen deprivation—the brain—was destroyed. Thus, a beating heart and spontaneous or artificially maintained respiration supported a senseless and unresponsive body for indefinite periods of time. This state was recognized early by the French neurologists who coined a term to describe it—*coma dépassé*. The condition was considered to be a supercoma in which even the vegetative functions were lost and from which recovery would not occur. The state might have attracted little notice had not the newly developed transplant surgery required well-perfused and viable organs. This focused the attention of the medical profession on the necessity to identify a body as dead when the brain became permanently devoid of function, so that healthy, well-irrigated organs might be obtained for transplantation.

Thus, a new concept was introduced into thanatology, namely, that death was cerebrally based and quite independent of cardiac and/or respiratory function (8,11). The incorporation of the concept of cerebral death into the philosophy of modern society did not introduce a second type of death, it simply brought into focus what had been implicitly assumed for years by physicians, philosophers and lawyers—that death occurred when the brain became permanently inactive, even though the signs of death were to be found in the absence of activity of the heart and lungs. Although these signs still heralded death in most persons, new criteria indicative of the irreparable loss of brain function had to be developed for the exceptional case in which they were not applicable.

The ideal criteria for the determination of cerebral death should have the following characteristics:

1. Be simple, uniform (the same for all types of cases), and interpretable by any physician,
2. Give unequivocal, not graded, results (475),
3. Be compatible with traditional methods of determining death,
4. Be acceptable to the general public,
5. Exclude reversible conditions that simulate death,
6. Assess several functions to minimize the chances of error (209).

Unfortunately, no set of criteria yet proposed has achieved these ideals.

Before discussing the specific criteria that have been suggested, some consideration should be given to the general principles to be used in the selection of the criteria and definition of the terms involved.

Obviously, the first point must be a definition of the endpoint—cerebral death. At the one extreme is the view that cerebral death represents the total and permanent destruction of the entire brain (475); at the other end is the psychosocial concept that cerebral death is the permanent loss of those functions that subserve human interactions (477).

It is understandable that physicians holding such diverse views would require different standards to establish cerebral death. In the present social climate, only a somatic concept of death seems acceptable to the general population; this discussion will therefore deal with sets of criteria related to loss of total brain function, as determined by standard clinical and/or laboratory examinations.

Principles For Determining Cerebral Death

The methods used to establish cerebral death may be divided into four categories:

I. Those examinations that are carried out before critical tests for cerebral death are applied and that are designed to identify any remediable condition which may be responsible for the patient's deathlike

state. These prerequisites include the trial of appropriate therapeutic measures for any treatable conditions. Only when these endeavors have failed should the specific tests for cerebral death be applied.
II. Those basic tests that are necessary to determine a cessation of cerebral function.
III. Those tests that are not ordinarily considered essential for the diagnosis of a dead brain, but which, if any of the results of examinations of the other categories have been equivocal, may give confirmatory evidence of absence of cerebral function.
IV. The period of time that the above findings must be present to assure permanence.

Prerequisites to the Application of Criteria for Cerebral Death

The transition from respiratory and cardiac indications of death to neurological criteria did not lessen the fears that reversible conditions mimicking the new criteria might be unrecognized. Physicians particularly aware of the many conditions—some lethal and some benign—that might cause deep coma devised screening tests that should be carried out before any criteria to certify brain death are applied. Because the characteristics of coma do not differentiate the reversible from the irreversible state, most clinicians have sought either by history or by clinical or laboratory examinations to determine the primary cause of the cerebral impairment and to instigate appropriate therapy. In fact, to ensure that a remediable condition will not be missed, some sets of criteria for cerebral death are only to be applied to suspects with a known, primary, irreparable condition of the brain, no matter how deeply unconscious or neurologically incapacitated the patients are.

No Evidence of Remediable Exo- or Endogenous Intoxication.   In many formulations of criteria of cerebral death, this prerequisite consists of the elimination of any possibility of drug intoxication. Although at the present time this is the most common cause of reversible deep and prolonged coma, many other remediable conditions have unconsciousness as their outstanding manifestation. A multitude of such exo- and endogenous factors are enumerated in textbooks (378). Dysfunctions of many organs, in particular the liver (hepatic coma), kidney (uremic coma) and pancreas (diabetes and hypoglycemia), are associated with deep coma that may be relieved by appropriate treatment. The clinical determination of these conditions may be easy when an adequate history is available, but without any knowledge of the precomatose state the diagnosis may require extensive laboratory examinations and even therapeutic testing. The level of glucose in the blood should be critically evaluated; abnormalities may represent pancreatic disease or hyperglycemia from damage to brainstem centers or from the intravenous administration of the glucose solutions in emergency treatment.

Difficulties in eliminating the possibility of drug intoxication arise from the unreliable history of drug ingestion, the virtual impossibility of obtaining accurate analyses of toxic agents within a few hours, and the assessment of the significance of minimal amounts of drugs in the blood. In the Collaborative Study, reports of drug levels in the blood were frequently delayed hours or days, and when obtained were often in the therapeutic range even though the patient was deeply comatose. Moreover, although the protocol required that blood be drawn in every case, half of the patients admitted to the study never had blood analyzed for intoxicants. These difficulties raise the question as to how reliable laboratory controls for drug intoxication actually are. These problems are not peculiar to cerebral death. In the control of pharmacological levels of anticonvulsive drugs, similar difficulties have been encountered.

Absence of Hypothermia.   Many of the historical cases of revival occurred in individuals who had been exposed for some hours to low environmental temperatures, often as the result of an alcoholic stupor. In such hibernating states, the blood pressure falls, the heart rate slows, the respiration is extremely shallow, and the cool cerebrum requires little metabolic energy. Such states are not confused with death when technical means are available to record an inaudible heart beat and detect neuronal activity.

Still, because hypothermia may be responsible for states resembling death, most criteria for the determination of cerebral death include the proviso that the body temperature must be in the normal range. In children, and particularly infants, this factor is crucial, for their temperatures are quite susceptible to environmental conditions.

Absence of Cardiovascular Shock.   In lesions involving the brainstem and hypothalamic centers, in addition to disturbances of thermal regulation, vasomotor control may be impaired and the blood pressure may fall to shock levels. If the blood pressure cannot be elevated, cardinal criteria of brain death may be invalidated, for a low blood pressure will suppress both cerebral blood flow and EEG activity, giving rise to a spurious impression of permanent cessation of cerebral functions.

Presence of an Irreparable Lesion. There is no doubt that the accuracy of diagnosis of cerebral death is enhanced if the criteria are applied only to those cases in which the causative factor is known to be an irreparable, organic intracranial lesion. Some authors (148) specify that this must be due to direct damage to the brain or increased intracranial pressure. Others (327) emphasize that the condition must be irreparable, and still others (399), believe that the cause of the coma and apnea must be established by personal contact with the subject and direct knowledge of the patient's history and medical findings. These conditions limit the application of criteria for cerebral death, since many people are brought into emergency rooms comatose and without a medical history or accompanying persons to provide such information. The difficulties in the clinical determination of an irreparable cerebral lesion in the emergency room may be insurmountable. The frequent combination of shock and respiratory embarrassment causes such overwhelming signs of neurological depression that a precise diagnosis is not possible before these conditions are successfully treated. Moreover, the exigencies of resuscitative measures often preclude the performance of examinations essential for an accurate early diagnosis.

Even after the vital functions have been restored to as normal a state as possible, the establishment of a definitive diagnosis—if the patient's condition has not been previously known or is not obvious—may require time-consuming examinations. If one of the common etiological states (myocardial infarction, cerebral trauma or intracranial vascular disease) is not apparent, the gamut of conditions producing coma must be explored, and a therapeutic test may be necessary to confirm the cause. Certainly, the possibility of the common treatable disorders, such as drug intoxication and intracranial hematomas, should be ruled out if the diagnosis is uncertain. This may require drug surveys, angiography, isotope scan, or computerized tomography. It is possible that, although the original primary condition was remediable, the brain may be dead as the result of anoxia due to complicating intracranial pressure. In these circumstances, a therapeutic test—as well as confirmatory examinations for cerebral death—is essential.

These preliminary requirements, in spite of their limitations and difficult accession, assure that the results of the application of specific criteria for cerebral death will not be misinterpreted.

Basic Criteria of Cerebral Death

The determination that the brain is dead is primarily based upon the clinical demonstration of deep coma, apnea and absence of the cephalic reflexes.

The unequivocal proof of these states is the cardinal indication of a dead brain; one or more of these defects may be associated with irreparable damage to the encephalon, but brain death requires that all three of them be present. To pronounce a brain dead when some degree of consciousness is present, spontaneous respiratory efforts are made even irregularly, or one or more of the cranial reflexes is active, is a perverted use of the term "brain death." The absence of both cerebral hemisphere and brainstem functions (manifested by lack of consciousness and respiration, respectively) is associated with a lethal outcome in 91% of cases. Yet, even in deep coma when no clinical manifestations of cerebral activity are apparent, other studies—electroencephalographic or metabolic—may indicate that the cerebrum still functions in part or in whole. In fact, electroencephalography demonstrates biological activity in about one-half of the population of comatose, apneic and moribund patients.

Although a very sensitive indicator of impaired brainstem function, apnea does not preclude the possibility that other functions mediated by the mesencephalon, pons and medulla oblongata may remain intact. Hence, to declare a brainstem nonfunctional, all its activities, particularly the cephalic reflexes, must be shown to be in abeyance. On the initial examination of the 459 unresponsive patients who died in the Collaborative Study (Table VIII–1), 141 individuals had some response in one or more cephalic reflexes. No one cephalic reflex was discriminative enough to identify all persons with preserved reflexes. The pupillary response to light came the closest, but it was present in only two thirds of the cases with viable brainstems. Nor does the size of the pupils provide an indication of the state of the brainstem, although dilated pupils are more commonly associated with other evidence of absent brainstem activity than are con-

Table VIII–1.   State of Cephalic Reflexes in 459 Moribund Patients of Collaborative Study Series at Initial Examination.

	Status of Reflex		
Reflex	Absence of reaction	Reaction present	Unable to examine
All cephalic	271	141	47
Pupillary (light)	367	90 (20)*	2
Corneal	385	72 (6)	2
Oculocephalic	399	53 (1)	7
Vestibular	364	56 (1)	39
Jaw jerk	401	36 (6)	22
Snout	422	23 (4)	14
Pharyngeal	368	22 (2)	69
Swallowing	363	21 (1)	75
Cough	377	20 (1)	62
Audio-ocular	444	5 (0)	10

*Numbers in parentheses indicate the cases with isolated preservation of the reflex.

stricted pupils. It is therefore apparent that although some cephalic reflexes are statistically more discriminating than others, and, in practice, more consistently tested, all cephalic reflexes should be examined to obtain the maximal accuracy. Combinations of 2, 3, or even 4 reflexes will not reveal the total function of the brainstem, although the percentage of activity undiagnosed may be under 3% and clinically of no significance (Table VIII–2).

Allen et al. (9) found that the combination of pupillary light, oculocephalic and vestibular reflexes had the greatest discriminative power; however, this combination would leave 4% of the comatose and apneic patients with one or more active reflexes. The reliability of other combinations of reflexes is shown in table VIII–2.

The prerequisites and clinical criteria, even if entirely met on one occasion, are not an absolute indication of a dead brain. The press of resuscitative activities in the Emergency Room or Intensive Care Unit often is responsible for the deliberate or accidental omission of certain routine neurological examinations of comatose and apneic patients. Technical difficulties may make procedures hazardous or impossible to accomplish. Commonly, the diagnostic workup is not complete. Because the patient has an obvious head injury, blood examinations for other reversible conditions such as drug ingestion, diabetes, etc., are not requested. Intratracheal tubes may make it impossible to examine pharyngeal or other cephalic reflexes. The electroencephalogram may contain so much artifactual material that it is impossible to interpret. Even if all tests have been meticulously performed, one or more may be equivocal. It has been argued that if physicians and laboratories could make accurate examinations there would be no difficulty in meeting prerequisites and criteria, but, unfortunately, that cannot always be achieved—not because of incompetence of the personnel, but because the exigencies of emergency treatment have a higher priority than extraneous diagnostic procedures. For these reasons,

Table VIII–2. Number of Missed Cases with Preserved Reflexes if State of Cephalic Reflexes Were Based Upon a Sample of Combinations of Cephalic Reflexes.

Combination of reflexes	Cases with active reflexes missed	
	Number	Percentage
Pupillary and corneal	29*	5.8%
Pupillary, corneal and oculocephalic	22	4.4%
Pupillary, corneal, oculocephalic and vestibular	18	3.6%
Pupillary, corneal, oculocephalic and jaw jerk	14	2.8%
Pupilliary, corneal and vestibular	19	3.8%
Pupillary, corneal and jaw jerk	15	3.0%
Pupillary, corneal, jaw jerk and vestibular	14	2.8%

*Of these, 11 had small pupils and 18 dilated pupils.

it is desirable to have, in addition to the usual clinical criteria, a means of establishing with finality the presence of a dead brain. Since this yardstick will determine death in a patient with no obvious chance of regaining a normal existence, the risks of the procedure may be somewhat greater than ordinarily considered acceptable for diagnostic tests. This added assurance may be obtained by prolonging the period of observation, or by the application of a test, independent of the basic criteria, that alone is capable of indicating the absence of brain function.

The disadvantage of overlong waiting has been previously discussed. A period of 6 hours after the ictus provides adequate time for all appropriate diagnostic and therapeutic procedures to be completed and for the cardiovascular system to stabilize. If organ transplantation is a consideration, a further delay increases the risk of cardiac arrest before cerebral death is pronounced and organs can be removed from a beating-heart cadaver.

Confirmatory Tests of Cerebral Death

In patients who meet the clinical criteria of cerebral death, confirmatory studies of the state of the brain are often needed to substantiate the diagnosis. These ancillary examinations are measurements of cerebral potentials, cerebral blood flow, cerebral metabolism and cerebral structure, each of which provides an independent estimate of the absence of cerebral function. The advantages, limitations and reliability of these examinations have been discussed in previous sections of this book. In tabular form they are displayed in Table VIII–3 along with references to the pages where a detailed account of each test may be found.

Many of the ancillary techniques used for the confirmation of cerebral death require operative procedures and intricate manipulations by highly skilled personnel which render them almost impossible to perform while resuscitative and diagnostic examinations are being carried out in the emergency room or intensive care unit. Many also require venous, arterial or cranial punctures, which, although of little risk in a normal person, may be hazardous in a seriously ill person. Consequently, these factors must be carefully considered in selecting the most appropriate confirmatory test(s) to be used in a case with a specific primary condition.

Temporal Factors in Determining Cerebral Death

Irrespective of the basis for the criteria of cerebral death, two temporal factors are of great importance: one, the time after the ictus that the standards are applied, and the other, the period during which the criteria must be met to assure that the alterations are permanent. The first consideration is limited in practice by a number of circumstances. The clinical and laboratory tests for cerebral death require some hours to perform. Emergency measures for basic life support can rarely be completed within 6 hours of the primary insult, since resuscitative measures are time-consuming and their effectiveness requires some hours to assess. In fact, in the Collaborative Study, the median time from insult to the beginning of the initial EEG was 8.4 hours; in only 5% of cases was the testing started within an hour of the ictus. Such a delay, allaying concern of relatives that a hasty decision is being made, may be advantageous. Because the main reason for an early determination of brain death is to obtain viable organs for transplantation, the propitious time for application of cerebral death criteria might be deduced from consideration of the natural course of individuals with ECS.

In the first six hours after a cerebral insult, there is only a small mortality, but from 6 to 12 hours the number of deaths increases steadily. Hence, to delay the determination of cerebral death for six hours would result in the loss of few potential donors, but after that time there would be a steady outfall. On the other hand, if the criteria were applied and met during the period of shock after the ictus, the spurious conclusion of cerebral death could deprive persons of the chance of resuscitation and revival. Based on these considerations, a lapse of six hours from the ictus may be considered an appropriate interval for resuscitative procedures and stabilization of vital functions. •

The time that the criteria should be operative is an unsettled question. Logically, the period of observation of the clinical phenomena should be sufficiently long that patients, misdiagnosed as being in irreparable states, may be identified by the return of brain function, the earliest evidence of which is reflex activity. An estimate of this period may be gained by consideration of the times at which comatose and apneic persons with unobtainable cephalic reflexes on initial examinations regained the responses. Some of the patients who eventually recovered their reflexes and survived showed no indication of recovery until 30 hours after the ictus (Table VIII–4). Hence, it would seem that if clinical findings alone are to be the criteria of death, an observation period of several days is necessary to identify all individuals who could recover. This period is so prolonged

Table VIII-3.   Ancillary Tests for Cerebral Death.

	Hours after Insult	Findings Indicative of Brain Death*	Reliability (percentage)	General Use
I. Related to brain potentials				
EEG (p. 81)	6+	ECS	99	++++
Depth recording (p. 91) ...	24+	ECS	99	+
Steady (DC) potentials (p. 93) ...	6+	Nasal = scalp potentials	Unknown(U)	+
Evoked potentials (p. 93) ...	6+	Absent	99	+++
II. Related to cerebral blood flow				
Quantitative CBF (p. 39) ...	12+	Less than 150 cc/min.	UU	+
Angiography—4 vessel (p. 41) ...	6+	No intracranial dye	99	++
Gamma camera scan (p. 45) ...	6+	Empty cranium	99	+++
Bolus (p. 46)	6+	No cephalic bolus	99	++++
EchEG—midline pulsation (p. 50)	1+	No midline pulsation	99	+
Isotope clearance—brain (p. 42) ...	24+	No clearance	U	+
—spinal (p. 43) ...	6+	No isotope in cranium	U	+
Ophthalmic artery retina (p. 53) ...	1+	Sludging	99	++++
angiography (p. 54) ...	6+	Persistent opacification	U	++
Fluorescein—arm-retina (p. 54) ...	1+	Greater than 30 seconds	U	++
Doppler flowmeter (p. 54) ...	1+	High systolic carotid flow absent or 0-0 orthodromic ophthalmic artery flow	U	+++
Intracranial pressure (p. 38) ...	12+	Equal or above systolic B.P.	U	+
Computerized tomography—Enhanced (p. 50) ...	1+	No intracranial vessels	U	+++
III. Related to cerebral metabolism				
$AVDO_2$ (p. 63)	6+	Less than 2 vol%	U	++
$CMRO_2$ (p. 61)	6+	Less than 1ml/gm/min	U	+++
CSF lactic acid (p. 63) ...	6+	More than 3 mg%	99	+
Brain temperature (p. 54) ...	24+	Less than 90°F	U	+
IV. Related to brain structure				
Computerized tomography (p. 50) ...	24+	Homogeneous density of brain	U	+++

*The findings indicative of a dead brain should be present for at least 30 minutes unless another ancillary test has demonstrated brain death for 30 minutes in which case a single examination is adequate.

Table VIII–4.   Time of Recovery of Initially Absent Cephalic Reflexes.

	Time of return of reflexes after Ictus	Moribund	Survivors
	Hours	Number of Cases	Number of Cases*
Second Examination	6	25	3
Third Examination	12	10	2
Fourth Examination	18	6	3
Fifth Examination	30	3	2
Sixth Examination	54	2	—
Seventh Examination	78	2	—
Total number of cases		48	10

*One additional surviving case had preserved cephalic reflexes at the first two examinations, then absent reflexes, with recovery again at subsequent examinations.

that 60% of apneic and comatose persons would have had cardiac arrest before they could be pronounced cerebrally dead.

The period of ECS after which recovery is impossible is not definitely established. Experimentally, ECS need be maintained only a few minutes by intracranial hypertension above systolic blood pressure to produce a permanent isoelectric state. However, in drug intoxications, isoelectric states have persisted for as long as two days with subsequent complete recovery (99, 141). For this reason, early writers recommended that ECS should be present at least 2–3 days before cerebral death was assumed. But as rapid methods to identify intoxicating agents became available, the time necessary to consider an isoelectric record as indicative of a permanent state was shortened to one day (34), 12 hours (327), 6 hours (469), 4 hours (233), 3 hours (135, 406), 30 minutes (148), and even 15 minutes (501). Although some patients in the Collaborative Study had a return of biological activity after ECS for 30 minutes, all normothermic and unintoxicated individuals with ECS had a cardiac arrest within a few days.

The duration of anoxia necessary to ensure a dead brain is no more definitely established. Neurophysiologists, basing their judgment on comparative studies, maintain that a few minutes of anoxia is sufficient under normal environmental states to produce a dead brain, but physicians, considering their clinical experience, believe that the time should be hours or days.

The literature provides various estimates of the minimal period of absence of CBF required to produce a dead brain. The German Surgical Society (148) stated that, in cases of head injury or intracranial hypertension, cerebral death may be assumed when the cerebral circulation has been arrested for 30 minutes. Tönnis and Frowein (460) concluded that a complete cessation of CBF for 30 minutes indicated a dead brain. On clinical evidence, Jorgensen et al. (221) concluded that 20 minutes was adequate. Prochazka (386) came to a similar conclusion. However, Waltregny (501) thought that a 15-minute absence of CBF was sufficient to establish cerebral death.

The times that the various criteria must be present to assure a dead brain differ greatly, and accordingly a universal limit is inappropriate. The period a given test must be applied to establish cerebral death may vary from a few minutes to 3 days.

Clinical Criteria of Cerebral Death

In spite of unresolved conceptual difficulties, many sets of criteria have been proposed in the scientific literature for the pronouncement of brain death. These formulae, usually evolved by consensus, were developed from certain preconceived concepts of cerebral death and were based upon clinical experience and retrospective analyses. Few were tested by prospective studies to determine their scope, i.e., the frequency with which patients suspected clinically of cerebral death meet such criteria, their accuracy, which is the reliability with which the criteria identify permanent lack of function of the brain, and their practicability in modern hospital settings. An attempt will be made to analyze the different categories in terms of these factors. Obviously, to examine individually all of the formulae which have been proposed in the last decade would be both time-consuming and repetitious. However, these sets of criteria may be grouped into five types, based upon the biomedical concept used in their formulation:

1. Clinical criteria per se
2. Clinical and EEG confirmatory tests
3. Clinical and cerebral blood flow comfirmatory tests
4. Clinical and metabolic confirmatory tests
5. Clinical and combinations of confirmatory tests.

Although the sets of criteria are classifiable into the above five groups, in some cases their categorization is somewhat arbitrary. Basically all groups rely upon clinical findings. However, even in the sets of clinical criteria, confirmatory tests are advocated under certain conditions to increase the degree of certainty.

Clinical Criteria per se.   For centuries, common law has placed the responsibility of determining death upon the physician but has not prescribed the means he should use to ascertain its presence. Even today the statutes regarding death merely state that "if in the opinion of a physician, based on ordinary standards of medical practice, there is absence of spontaneous respiration and cardiac function, death will have occurred at the time these functions ceased." No stipulations are made as to how the physician shall determine that spontaneous respiration and cardiac function have ceased— the only decree is that they shall be based on ordinary standards of medical practice. It is then natural that the clinician, when legally given the right to declare death on the basis of absence of brain function, should turn to clinical practices used in examination of the nervous system for determination of the absence of cerebral activity. Thus, these physicians believe that if reasonable attempts at resuscitation have failed, the absence of clinical manifestations of cerebral and brainstem functions meet the legal requirements to declare a brain dead, especially if these signs are present for 12 to 24 hours. This would seem to follow the common practice hallowed by medical tradition.

Physicians agree, in general, that the clinical criteria for the determination of cerebral death should relate to three principle considerations:

1. the absence of cerebral functions,
2. the absence of brainstem functions including respiration,
3. the permanency of these states.

The techniques used to determine that these criteria are met vary with the different sets of guidelines, and will probably change as new diagnostic procedures are developed to measure brain activity.

In most sets of criteria based upon clinical findings certain prerequisites are specified to insure that reversible causes of coma and apnea have been identified, and, if present, adequately treated. This provision is very difficult if not impossible to meet in some cases in which a clinical diagnosis is not evident. Multiple laboratory examinations and even therapeutic tests may be necessary to establish the cause of the coma and apnea. Of course, if the physician has had long professional contact with the patient and knows the causative condition to be incurable, his clinical judgment may adequately meet this prerequisite.

Although the Harvard criteria are sometimes said to be based solely upon clinical tests, they do include a confirmatory EEG and for this reason, they are not used as the prototype for clinical criteria of cerebral death. The standards proposed by Mohandas and Chow (327) of the University of Minnesota ("Minnesota Criteria") will be considered the prototype, although the recent proposal by the Working Party of Great Britain and Northern Ireland (517) is more clearly defined. These formulae have the attractive advantage that no laboratory techniques are required, although quite complicated examinations may be necessary to establish the prerequisite that the primary lesion be known to be an irreparable destruction of the brain.

Using the data bank of the Collaborative Study, the diagnostic categories of cerebral trauma, cerebrovascular disease, CNS infection and cerebral neoplasm are assumed to meet the basic prerequisite of the Minnesota Criteria (Table VIII–5). In these categories, there were a total of 273 cases, of which 180 cases met the three criteria on one occasion; however,

Table VIII–5.   Minnesota Criteria.

Prerequisite: Irreparable intracranial lesion
   Criteria: No spontaneous movement
   Apnea when off respirator for 4 minutes
   Absent brainstem reflexes—dilated and fixed pupils, absent corneal, ciliospinal, doll's head phenomenon, gag, vestibular, and tonic neck reflexes
   Duration: 12 hours

Table VIII–6.   Criteria of Cerebral Death Based on Clinical Concepts.

Author or Other Test	Criteria in Addition to Coma and Apnea			Confirmatory Tests
	Prerequisite	Reflexes	Time	
Beecher[34]	No hyperthermia nor drugs	Absent reflexes	24 hours	EEG
Mohandas and Chow[327]	Known irreparable organic encephalopathy	Cephalic reflexes absent	12 hours	
Royal Colleges[399]	No depressent or blocking drugs Normothermia Metabolic disturbances excluded Irremediable structural brain damage established	Brainstem reflexes absent Pupils fixed and unresponsive No corneal Vestibulo-ocular absent No gag reflex No motor brainstem response No respiratory effort after disconnection	24 hours EEG, if available	
Minnesota Med. Assn[104]	Reversible CNS dysfunction excluded (T below 90 F or intoxication)	Cerebral unresponsivity Absent brainstem reflexes Pupils greater than 5 mm and fixed	12 hours	
Working Party G.B.[517]	Irremediable structural brain damage	Apneic coma (No respiration with $PaCO_2 > 50$ mm Hg) Brainstem reflexes absent	Unspecified	Independent certification by 2 physicians

17 patients had biological activity in the EEG at that time. Although 141 individuals met all three criteria for a period of 12 hours, 11 of these did not have ECS at either the initial or 12-hour examination. Hence, if cerebral death was diagnosed on the basis of these criteria, 8% of the patients would have had resuscitative efforts stopped while the EEG still had evidence of cerebral electrical activity. Nonetheless, the criteria, if met, *predicted* a dying or moribund, but not necessarily dead, brain. One would conclude that the accuracy of these criteria in defining a nonfunctioning brain is 92% and the scope is 67%.

Such criteria of death are open to several criticisms (Table VIII–6). In the first place, although the clinical manifestations of absence of brain function are adequate to identify moribund patients, they fail to recognize neuronal activity that may be demonstrated by electroencephalography or metabolic examinations. Thus, approximately 10% of persons meeting these clinical criteria of cerebral death have biological activity in their electroencephalograms. Is the diagnosis of cerebral death justifiable under these circumstances? One may argue that fluctuating electrical potentials do not constitute human life. However, such considerations lead to imponderable questions bordering euthanasia that should not be a part of death decisions at this point in time.

A second criticism may be directed at the length of time these criteria should be present. As discussed previously, if clinical findings alone are the criteria of death, several days of observation would be necessary to allow sufficient time for all individuals who might recover to exhibit signs of revival.

Clinical Criteria and Confirmatory Tests

Although a few sets of clinical criteria did not require any confirmatory tests, most authors or committees considered that a second examination should be made to verify the diagnosis of cerebral death. In most cases this consisted of an EEG so that an objective record would be available. However, whether or not such an examination was made, sometimes was left to the judgment of the attending physician, and sometimes made mandatory.

Optional EEG confirmatory test.   Some doubts as to the reliability of the clinical criteria to establish a dead brain seem to have arisen in the minds of physicians, for the option of electroencephalographic confirmation is frequently mentioned in discussing the diagnosis of cerebral death. Rarely, however, are guidelines given as to the cases in which this option should be exercised. In the recommendations of the prestigious Harvard Committee on Irreversible Coma*, it is stated that an isoelectric EEG is a valuable confirmatory test. The other criteria required (Table VIII–7) are quite restrictive and limit the number of comatose and apneic persons who might be declared brain dead.

If these clinical criteria are used alone as a basis for a decision of cerebral death, and applied to the Collaborative Study data bank, only 32 patients of the 442 cases meeting the prerequisites fulfilled all criteria for 24 hours. Of these moribund individuals, 13 never had a flat EEG so that with the confirmatory test, only 19 (4%) of the original population at risk could meet the Harvard criteria for irreversible coma. Obviously, these requirements are too stringent for practical use.

The Harvard criteria have served as a model for a number of sets of criteria for cerebral death, the details of which differ only in minor respects. The slight changes introduced have related to the advisability of including the spinal reflexes, of adding a criterion related to a failing cardiovascular system and of shortening the time required.

The absence of the spinal reflexes as a criterion was questioned early, since it was obvious that the brain might be dead while spinal cord functions persisted. Moreover, the presence or absence of the spinal reflexes was admitted to depend upon the regression or persistence of spinal shock. Accordingly, their exclusion was advised by European and American writers, and even by members of the Harvard Committee (36).

Mandatory EEG confirmatory test.   That a comatose and apneic patient might be shown to have a dead brain by the demonstration of absence of cortical electrical potentials was suggested in 1959 by Fischgold and Mathis (135) who described the EEG changes associated with states of impaired consciousness and the flat record that developed as death approached. Schwab and his associates in several papers (398, 419) emphasized the value of EEG in the determination of brain death. But it was the report of the Americn Electroencephalographic Society's Ad Hoc Committee on EEG Criteria for the Determination of Cerebral Death, based on a survey of American electroencephalographers and a review of French and Ger-

---

* The committee apparently considered "irreversible coma" as synonymous with the brain death syndrome. However, as the term is often used in medical parlance, it refers to many comatose states that are often not closely nor necessarily related to death (252). These different connotations have given rise to misunderstandings. In this discussion of the Harvard Criteria the term will be considered to mean brain death. Elsewhere, it will have its usual connotation of a comatose existence.

Table VIII–7.   Harvard Criteria[34].

Prerequisite:	Absence of hypothermia and drug intoxication
Criteria:	Unresponsive coma
	Apnea
	Absent reflexes
Confirmation:	Isoelectric electroencephalogram
Duration:	24 hours

man literature on the subject, that established the reliability of the EEG for the diagnosis of a dead brain. The report stated that the only survivors after a verifiable ECS among 1,665 cases of isoelectric cerebral death suspects were persons suffering from drug intoxication, and concluded: "Neither the neurological characteristics of *coma dépassé* alone, nor electrocerebral silence by itself is a certain indication of cerebral death, but together they constitute strong presumptive evidence that such is the case, provided that depressant drugs in anesthetic levels as a cause are eliminated (431).

The requirements advocated by Schwab et al.(398, 419) may be accepted as the prototype of this set of criteria (Table VIII–8). If these standards are applied to the Collaborative Study series, 442 patients would meet the prerequisites, and of these, 185 had ECS on their initial EEG record. However, the requirement that all criteria be absent for 24 hours eliminates all but 19 cases, the same number that met the Harvard criteria.

If the requirements were modified so that only the cephalic reflexes had to be absent, 278 persons would qualify on the first examination and 144 of these (51.8%) would have ECS on the initial examination. Since all would die, the accuracy for a dead brain on only one examination would be 100%.

These critera have been used frequently with slight modifications to simplify the tests or to shorten the time of application (Table VIII-9). The Japanese Collaborative Study adopted criteria that illustrate this principle

Table VIII–8.   Schwab's Criteria.

Prerequisite:	None
Criteria:	Apnea
	Total areflexia
	Dilated and fixed pupils
	No change in pulse rate with eyeball pressure
	Flat EEG for 30 minutes recording with interelectrode resistance greater than 50,00 ohms
	No auditory evoked potentials
Duration:	30 minutes (later, 24 hours[333])

Table VIII–9.   Japanese Study Criteria.

Prerequisite:	Gross primary brain lesion
Criteria:	Deep coma
	Apnea
	Bilateral dilated pupils
	Absent pupillary and corneal reflexes
	Isoelectric electroencephalogram
	40 mm Hg fall in blood pressure with persistent hypotension
Duration:	6 hours

(469). They have required that the pathology be a gross primary brain lesion. Then their criteria are: coma, apnea, dilated fixed pupils and absent corneal reflexes, an isoelectric EEG, and a test for the autonomic state, namely, that there be a drop in blood pressure, a factor mentioned originally by Mollaret(330) but rarely included in sets of criteria later (Table VIII–10).

If these criteria are applied to the Collaborative Study data, in the categories of cerebral trauma, cerebral vascular disease, infections of the brain, and brain tumors, there were 273 cases. Only 11 cases (4% of the selected population) met all the Japanese Study criteria, including hypotension, for 6 hours.

Obviously, the use of vasopressor drugs to maintain the circulation, although employed in only 20% of the cases in the Collaborative Study, compromised the statistical evaluation of the Japanese criteria. One would conclude that the Japanese criteria applied to cases as managed in the U.S.A. would have extremely limited applicability, for only 4% of the population meeting entrance conditions could qualify as cerebrally dead. However, if the requirement of a fall of 40 mm Hg in blood pressure is omitted, the scope is expanded to 36 patients who had a BP below 80 mm Hg for 6 hours, and if the hypotensive criterion is also eliminated, 164 patients meet the remaining Japanese Study Criteria.

Clinical EEG and Cerebral Blood Flow Criteria.   In *coma dépassé,* Wertheimer et al. (510) recognized that the cerebral circulation was absent. Subsequent clinical and experimental studies convinced many European neurologists and neurosurgeons that cerebral death is the result of a total infarction of the brain. The mechanism is complicated (see p. 38), but the end result is cessation of the cerebral blood flow. With this concept of the pathogenesis of cerebral death, it was natural that clinicians should consider the demonstration of cessation of intracranial circulation as evidence of a dead brain in a comatose and apneic individual without cephalic reflexes. Accordingly, many European investigators, especially the Swedish (who have contributed so much to the knowledge of CBF), added to

Table VIII–10. Criteria of Cerebral Death Based on Clinical and Electroencephalographic Criteria.

Author or Organization	Criteria in Addition to Coma and Apnea				Confirmatory or Other Test
	Prerequisites	Reflexes	EEG	Time applicable	
Alderete et al[6]	Normothermia No drugs	Areflexia	ECS	24 hours	
Allegheny county[8]		Areflexia	ECS	2 hours	
Barnard[515]	Normothermia Treatment ineffective	Pupils fixed and dilated	ECS	1 hour	EKG flat 1 hour
Berkutov et al[45]	Brain trauma	Corneal and pupillary reflexes absent	ECS	2 hours	
Canadian Medical Association[86]	Normothermia No drugs	Areflexia	ECS	24 hours	
CIOMS[101]	Normothermia No drugs Not infant	Areflexia	ECS	—	BP failing
Cooley[492]	None	Cephalic areflexia	ECS	—	BP failing
German Surgical Society[148]	Brain trauma or ICP	Pupils dilated and fixed	ECS 1 hour	12 hours	Or angio. proof of no CBF for 30 min.
Ivan[211]	No remedial condition	Cephalic areflexia	ECS	6 hours	BP failing
Käufer and Penin[233]	None	Areflexia dilated pupils	ECS	4 hours	
Lorenz[296]	Diagnosis known	Areflexia	ECS	24 hours	Atropine 1 mg, without tachycardia
NCOP	History known	Areflexia dilated pupils	ECS	—	BP failing
Schwab[419]	Normothermia No drugs Electrolytes normal	Areflexia	ECS	24–72 hours	No change in pulse rate with ocular or carotid pressure
Solnitzky[443]	—	Cephalic areflexia	ECS	—	Angiography
Spann[444]	Normal electrolytes	Areflexia	ECS	6 hours	BP failing
U.S. Navy[472]	Diagnosis known No drugs Normothermia	Cephalic areflexia	ECS if possible	13 hours	
Waltregny et al[501]	—	Irreversible coma	ECS no depth activity	15 minutes	
Wawersik[503]	—	Pupillary areflexia	ECS	12 hours	Or no CBF for 30 minutes

the basic criteria the angiographic proof of circulatory arrest in the brain. These criteria are attractive because (a) they require a minimal time lapse between serious consideration of brain death and the establishment of an absent cerebral circulation, and (b) taken collectively, they are independent of etiology, including toxic agents (208) (Table VIII–11).

Unfortunately, these criteria could not be tested against the Collaborative Study series, because, although a majority of cases in the study had primary intracerebral pathology which might have warranted diagnostic angiographic studies, only 17 angiograms were performed. However, other studies have shown a high correlation between clinical and EEG evidence of lack of brain function and angiographic non-filling of cerebral vessels. (30, 70, 77, 97, 164, 272, 485)

The state of the cerebral circulation complements the clinical impression of brain death in several respects. First, this measurement offers a means of establishing brain death irrespective of etiology, for a thirty-minute cessation of CBF from any cause predicates a dead brain. Secondly, because a long wait for laboratory determinations is unnecessary, an early diagnosis of brain death provides more viable donor organs for transplantation. Thirdly, in situations where medicolegal questions may arise, such as organ transplantation, it is wise to have more than one means of confirming brain death.

Metabolic confirmatory tests.   Obviously in death, the encephalon does not use oxygen (O_2), so that the demonstration of zero or near zero cerebral O_2 consumption should constitute evidence of a dead brain. However, the techniques for the determination of cerebral metabolism are so complicated that they can be carried out only in research units. Moreover, because they depend upon the quantitative measurement of CBF, which in cases of cerebral death has many sources of error (p. 61), the results are quite variable, even when technical difficulties encountered in obtaining venous blood from the jugular bulb and arterial blood samples in seriously ill patients are overcome. Consequently, $CMRO_2$ and $AVDO_2$ determinations, although of research interest, at this time have limited value in the routine determination of cerebral death. The high lactic acid content of

Table VIII–11.   Scandinavian Criteria.

Prerequisite:	None
Criteria:	Unresponsive coma
	Apnea
	Absence of cerebral functions, including brainstem reflexes
	Isoelectric encephalogram
	Nonfilling of cerebral vessels on 2 angiograms 25 minutes apart
Duration:	25 minutes

the cerebrospinal fluid should be a valid indicator of absence of normal cerebral metabolism. However, many physicians are loathe to do a spinal puncture and remove CSF on a patient with a foramen magnum block. As a result, this technique has not been sufficiently used to assess its value in determining cerebral death.

Combinations of confirmatory tests. The absence of CBF as determined by four vessel angiography is perhaps the most sensitive of the commonly used tests for a dead brain. However, because it is invasive, requires the injection of dye in vessels with a slow circulation and has the risk of technical complications, some clinicians consider that contrast angiography is impractical for routine use on patients hovering between life and death, and seek less traumatic, simpler, and yet, reliable means of determining death of the brain.

The members participating in the Collaborative Study sought to develop a formula whereby, using simple and non-invasive tests, the time of observation could be cut to a minimum. Within limits, the shorter the period of observation, the more individuals might be diagnosed as cerebrally dead, but if the interval was too brief, persons with dormant brains could not be distinguished from those with dead brains.

It was apparent that a diagnosis of cerebral death could not be made on the basis of a criterion related to a single functional system at any one point in time. A single clinical examination, EEG examination, or even cerebral blood flow determination fell short of an absolute diagnosis of cerebral death. Repetitive studies of a single functional system provide greater confidence, but, in some cases, the time periods are long, and many patients would die of cardiac arrest before they would meet the criteria. It seemed that a combination of the available determinants of cerebral death with particular attention to their simplicity and reliability would furnish the most practical solution to a quick and accurate diagnosis (Table VIII–12).

In the formula developed by the Collaborative Study, a six hour delay after the ictus was mandatory before the tests for cerebral death could be applied (99). This allowed sufficient time for appropriate diagnostic and therapeutic procedures to be carried out and for the cardiovascular system to stabilize. Then, with the patient under normal thermal and vascular conditions, the following standards had to be met for one-half hour:

1. Coma with cerebral unresponsiveness
2. Apnea
3. Absent cephalic reflexes and dilated pupils
4. Electrocerebral silence.

Table VIII–12.   Criteria of Cerebral Death Based on Multiple Tests.

Author of organization	Criteria in Addition to Coma and Apnea				Time applicable	Confirmatory or other test
	Prerequisites	Reflexes	EEG	CBF		
Crafoord[103]	Known history	Areflexia	ECS	Absent 10–15 minutes		
Bushart and Rittmeyer[81]	None	Areflexia	ECS	Absent by angiography	3 days	No DC potentials
Kramer[263]	Experienced neurologist consultant	Clinical diagnosis of CD	ECS	No CBF	—	Pulse rate unchanged after atropine
Netherlands RC Society[345]	—	Cephalic areflexia	ECS	No CBF by angiography, scintography or fluorescein retinography	—	No depth potentials
Walker[492]	—	Cephalic areflexia	ECS	No CBF by angiography	—	CMRO$_2$-low No depth potentials

If any of these criteria were equivocally met, the diagnosis had to be validated by the demonstration of absence of cerebral blood flow using a simple, minimally traumatic and reliable technique. A number of such methods are available. Which one is selected for a particular patient will depend upon the local conditions, facilities available, and the preferences of the attending physician. All are reliable in experienced hands. The most commonly used techniques include isotope angiography with the gamma camera (p. 45), echoencephalographic demonstration of the midline pulsations (p. 46), cerebral isotope bolus (p. 46) ophthalmoscopic examinations for sludging (p. 53), and enhanced CT (p. 50, Fig. VIII–1).

This formula provides for the rapid establishment of a dead brain and allows ancillary procedures to confirm this state if the criteria, as so often happens, are not completely met. Thus, if some diagnostic tests are unavailable, such as a survey for drugs, if the pupils are small, or, if the EEG is obscured by artifact, the diagnosis of a dead brain may be established by any technique demonstrating the absence of cerebral blood flow for 30 minutes.

Although the period of objective demonstration of complete lack of brain function is only 30 minutes, it would seem likely that if the tests were met, the deprivation would have been present for at least the previous six hours required for the preliminary diagnostic and therapeutic procedures to be performed. Hence, although a half-hour alone may be adequate as the extreme limit of human cerebral tolerance of anoxia, in all probability the proposed six hour delay would allow a very significant margin for error.

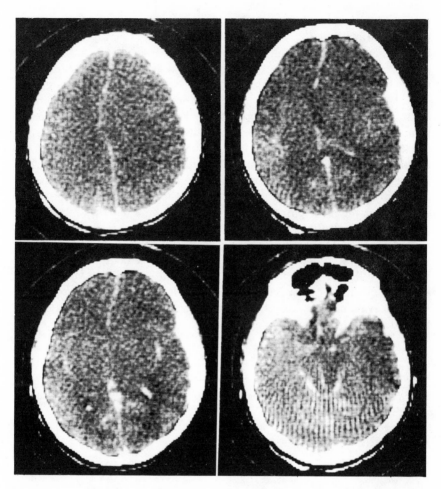

Fig. VIII–1.   Computerized tomograms to show the relatively homogenous appearance of a cerebrally dead brain. Note the absence of the ventricles and blood in the ambient cisterns, Sylvian fissures, and the right frontal subdural and/or extradural hematoma. The patient, a 19-year-old boy who had sustained multiple cranial fractures in a head-on auto collision, had both clinical and electroencephalographic evidence of cerebral death.

A General Formula for Cerebral Death

Each set of criteria, irrespective of the concept upon which it is based, is quite predictive of an existing or eventual brain death. However, some have restrictions that would unduly limit the number of comatose, apneic and moribund patients who could qualify. Some require such long periods of observation that the majority of suspects would have cardiac arrest before they could be declared dead. Many include certain prerequisites such as a known irreparable cause for the coma, which are often impossible to establish without special facilities. Moreover, in addition to a clinical neurological examination, they require confirmatory tests that use complex equipment not available in many smaller hospitals. Under these circumstances, the determination of death would have to be made upon cardiac arrest, or, solely, upon the clinical manifestations of cerebral death. To avoid this dilemma, doctors in small hospitals often transfer comatose and apneic patients to larger institutions as organ donors with the presumptive diagnosis of a dead brain. Not infrequently, such recipient hospitals, upon accepting an unknown case for organ transplant, have had the embarrassing experience to find that some of these transfer patients are neither afflicted with irreparable lesions nor brain dead.

It is, however, possible to make an accurate prediction of death due, with a high degree of certainty, to a dead brain in any hospital with their available facilities. The variable determinant is time. The fewer specialized facilities available, the longer the time required to establish that the brain is dead.

Table VIII–13.   Algorithm for Cerebral Death in Adults.

The patient, normothermic and normotensive[1], must be comatose, apneic and without cephalic reflexes, **and**

meet the conditions specified in A, B, or C.

A   1. This state must be present for at least 3 days, **or**

B   1. The primary condition must be known to be an irreparable lesion of the brain, **and**

    2. The patient, by appropriate examinations, must be shown to have for at least 30 minutes:
      a) electrocerebral silence in the EEG, **or**
      b) absence of cerebral blood flow[2], **or**

C   1. The primary condition, not a known irreparable lesion of the brain, has not responded to appropriate treatment, **and**

    2. The patient's EEG must be isoelectric for 2 days, **or**

    at least 6 hours after the ictus, the EEG must be isoelectric for 30 minutes and there must be no evidence of cerebral blood flow for 30 minutes.

---

[1] The rectal temperature should be above 90° F (32° C) and the systolic blood pressure should be above 80 mm Hg for hypothermia and hypopiesia may so depress cerebral activity that areflexia and ECS result; if these vital functions cannot be restored to a normal level, cerebral death may be declared on the basis of the other criteria and the absence of cerebral blood flow for 30 minutes.

[2] This may be determined by quantitative measurements of CBF, enhanced CT, four vessel angiography, cephalic passage of an isotope bolus intravenously injected, or demonstration of the absence of a midline echo.

In Table VIII–13 is an algorithm for the determination of cerebral death that can be used in any hospital. Criteria for cerebral death can be selected that are appropriate to the available facilities and will establish a dead brain within a maximal period of three days after the criteria are met. The weakest point in this formula is the demonstration of the total absence of the cephalic reflexes. In practice, one or more reflexes are often not examined or have equivocal findings so that the primary criterion cannot be met. It should be noted that persons meeting the "A" option, although all moribund, have approximately a 9% chance of having some activity in their EEGs, so that strictly speaking, only 91% of the individuals in this group have a dead brain. In the other two option groups, all persons meeting the criteria are cerebrally dead.

Because only approximately 26% of the patients meeting the primary criterion will survive more than 3 days, if organs are to be taken for transplant from a patient in a hospital where "A" criteria must be used, it would seem desirable to transfer the patients to a major medical center where the tests required in options "B" or "C" could be applied early.

These tests are applicable to adults; whether they are valid for young children and infants for whom criteria for cerebral death are less well established, is uncertain. For this reason, they are recommended only for use in adults.

Criteria of Brain Death in Infants and Children

It is commonly accepted that babies' brains are more resistant to anoxia and ischemia than adults' brains. This is based upon the lower $CMRO_2$ requirements of infants and the fact that the fontanelles and suture lines are open so that moderate changes in intracranial pressure are readily compensated. However, the blood pressure and perfusion pressures of infants and children are lower than in adults. Perhaps this explains the higher mortality from circulatory arrest in infants under one month of age than in other age groups (p 0.01), which Pampiglione et al. (364) reported.

In general, pediatricians have based a diagnosis of brain death on the same clinical criteria used for adults. However, the time that the criteria must be met has been less well defined, and various confirmatory tests have been advocated. Ashwal et al. (27) consider that if the clinical criteria—absence of spontaneous respiration, cranial reflexes and responsivity—are met, an isoelectric EEG and absence of CBF for a period of 30 minutes are evidence that a child's brain is dead. They believe that these criteria should be fulfulled for 24 hours in infants and neonates. Jährig

(214) considers the signs of brain death to be unresponsive coma, apnea, no response to trachael irritation through the intratrachael tube and a blood pressure below 30 mm Hg, which he believes indicates absence of cerebral perfusion. If uncertainty exists, ancillary tests for CBF may be used to confirm the diagnosis. Although body temperature has been advocated as a criterion (12), Jährig does not consider it a reliable indicator of a dead brain. Kero et al. (240) have suggested that the decreased variation in heart rate might be used as a sign of cerebral death.

Chapter IX

Legal Aspects of Cerebral Death

Introduction

A legal definition of death related to pulmonary and cardiac stoppage would seem to be medically outmoded, for resuscitative measures may restore the action of the heart and lungs but leave the subject inert with all the neurological characteristics of death. A more realistic definition might be cast in terms of the activity of the brain, which, after all, is the organ now medically considered to determine whether a person is alive or dead. The law, once new concepts are medically accepted, incorporates them into social codes. In the case of cerebral basis for death, its integration into the laws of the land has been hastened by a number of factors:

1. The need for early removal of organs for transplantation. If cardiac arrest was used as the criterion of death, the donor organs underwent such deterioration that their immunological reception by the recipient was poor at best. Although hypothermia or local perfusion of the donor organs decreased the likelihood of degradation, an organ from a beating-heart cadaver offered the best chance of a successful transplant.
2. The cost of prolonged use of extraordinary measures. The expense of resuscitative efforts in terms of money, professional personnel and hospital facilities made it imperative that their unnecessary use be eliminated.
3. The prolongation of sorrow and grief. Relatives, friends and business associates of the patient complained of the inhumanity of extended life-support measures, especially when the futility of the mechanical procedures became apparent to all.

4. The increasing awareness of the "right to die with dignity." Although some patients, at the time resuscitative measures are instituted, are legally disabled—either not of legal age, incompetent, or medically incapable of informed consent—many persons, aware of the indignities involved and still capable of informed consent, have requested that extraordinary measures not be applied if death is inevitable; or that if such measures have been introduced, they be discontinued so that death may proceed with dignity. On this basis, the next of kin, having been instructed in the legal requirements of informed consent, could request that further treatment be discontinued. (The court decisions have been somewhat varied depending upon such factors as the primary condition, age, religion and socioeconomic condition of the patient.)

With the brain as a basis for the declaration of death, it was perhaps natural that the legal profession selected the electroencephalogram as an objective measure of cerebral function. Thus, a flat electroencephalogram was thought to be a reliable and accurate objective method of establishing a dead brain.

However, the declaration of brain death solely on the basis of a flat EEG encountered a number of medical and legal obstacles. Almost from the beginning, the proposition that a flat EEG represented cerebral death was contested by both neurologists and electroencephalographers. They considered a flat EEG as evidence only of absence of activity in the cerebral hemispheres and not in the brainstem, which might still be sustaining respiration and the blood pressure. In fact, a flat EEG might not be conclusive evidence of even "cerebral" death, for numerous patients with drug intoxication were reported to have flat EEGs for over 24 hours, and yet, with appropriate therapy, they recovered (499). Moreover, electroencephalographers, realizing the difficulty of recording in emergency rooms and intensive care units, admitted that artifactual material and extracerebral potentials—e.g., EKG—often made the determination of a flat EEG difficult or impossible. For these reasons, most electroencephalographers were unwilling to declare a brain dead solely on the basis of a routine 30-minute flat electroencephalographic record (431). Accordingly, the initial, almost blind, reliance upon electroencephalography became tempered as experience accumulated.

Case Law Regarding Cerebral Death

The concept of cerebral or brain death as representing finite death has received support from a number of judicial decisions. These cases, in general, have related to the cause of death of individuals, cerebrally dead as the result of a criminal assault, from whom organs have been removed. In 1971, a jury in Portland, Oregon, had to decide on the cause of death of a man. He was comatose, with a flat EEG and mechanically ventilated as a result of a bullet wound, and his kidneys were removed for transplantation. Was it removal of the organs or the missile injury that caused death? The jury considered the bullet wound to be the proximate cause of death and found the assailant guilty of second-degree murder (185).

A year later, a jury in Virginia heard evidence regarding a suit against physicians for removing a heart while the donor, who met the criteria of cerebral death, was alleged to be still alive. The judge instructed the jury that they might use complete and irreversible loss of all function of the brain as a possible definition of death. The verdict was in favor of the defendants, and presumably was based upon the conclusion that death occurred when the brain ceased functioning and not when cardiac and respiratory activities stopped (185).

Two cases in California, in which the defense rested upon the claim that the accused assailants had not killed their victims because the heart was beating when removed for transplant, were decided with initially contrasting results (185). In one case, the judge instructed the jury to accept irreversible cessation of brain function as evidence of death; the accused was convicted of voluntary manslaughter. In the other case, the judge upheld the traditional definition of death and dismissed the manslaughter charge, but the decision was later reversed.

Another case was described in *Time Magazine* (June 7, 1976). The victim, struck over the head with a baseball bat, was comatose, apneic and had a flat EEG. After 7 days, mechanical resuscitative aids were discontinued. The defense for the assailant argued that the victim was not dead until the machines were disconnected, and hence the accused could not be convicted of murder. However, the judge instructed the Boston jury that, although brain death was not statutorily defined in Massachusetts, it (the jury) could construe brain death as legal death (348).

These case reports, and others with complicated conditions, (16,17) illustrate the difficulties which may be averted by the statutory recognition of brain death. Otherwise, extenuating circumstances may permit an assailant to contend that it was the removal of life support, and not the assault, that caused death. Even when there may be no criminal liability involved, families and physicians in states that do not have laws recognizing cerebral death encounter difficulties in donating organs for transplantation. Such an issue arose in the case of a 14-year-old girl who was seriously injured while riding her bicycle near Boston. Within a few days, she was found to be in irreversible coma, meeting all the criteria of cerebral death, including ECS and absence of cerebral circulation as demonstrated by bilateral carotid angiograms. Her parents wished to have her organs removed for transplantation while they were still in a good state of preservation and likely to be accepted in a recipient. A Superior Court Judge had to be petitioned to sanction the removal of the mechanical apparatus that kept the girl's heart and lungs functioning. In a precedent-setting ruling, the jurist declared that the child was, in fact, medically and legally dead, so all resuscitation might be stopped and the organs removed (347).

Statutory Definitions of Brain Death.   The need for a new basis for the determination of death came from the development of mechanical substitutes for respiratory and cardiac function, but the necessity for its legal recognition stemmed from the desire to identify the moment of death early, so that viable organs might be removed for transplantation. The first brain death statutes, enacted in Kansas, Maryland, Virginia and New Mexico (later in Oregon), provided alternative definitions for death. According to these laws, a person will be considered dead if, in the physician's opinion, based on ordinary standards of medical practice, there is either absence of function of the heart or of the brain, provided various qualifying criteria have been met—for example, that "attempts at resuscitation are considered hopeless," that "all therapeutic measures have been carried out," and that "the person is known to have an irreparable condition."

This dual definition was criticized, in particular by Capron and Kass, (87) because the statute implied that there were two concepts of death, either one of which, if satisfactorily met, would affirm the demise of the individual. Hence, in a particular case the physician must decide which criterion he will use; other physicians or jurists, reviewing the case, might conclude that a different basis for the decision would be more appropriate.

Such double standards might cause inconsistencies in the determination of the moment of death for purposes of inheritance. Not only does the time of death differ depending upon whether cardiac or brain criteria are used, but the duration of resuscitative measures may be influenced by the criterion to be applied. Moreover, there is the macabre situation of a person being considered dead for one purpose (such as transplantation of body organs) but alive for another (such as inheritance) if different definitions of death are used.

Because of these discrepancies, Capron and Kass proposed the following definition:

A person will be considered dead if in the announced opinion of a physician, based on ordinary standards of medical practice, he has experienced an irreversible cessation of spontaneous respiratory and circulatory functions. In the event that these functions have ceased, a person will be considered dead if in the announced opinion of a physician, based on ordinary standards of medical practice, he has experienced an irreversible cessation of spontaneous brain functions. Death will have occurred at the time when the relevant functions ceased.

A number of states have based statutes on this definition. Under these laws a person may be pronounced dead if there is irreversible cessation of spontaneous respiratory and cardiac funtion based on ordinary standards of medical practice. If these functions are being artificially maintained, the person may be declared dead if "no spontaneous brain function" (Alaska), "irreversible cessation of spontaneous brain functions" (Iowa, Michigan and West Virginia), "irreversible total cessation of brain function" (Louisiana), or "irreversible cessation of vital brain functions" (New Jersey) can be demonstrated by ordinary methods of medical practice.

Later statutory definitions of death have only specified that death is "irreversible cessation of total brain function, according to the usual and customary standards of medical practice" (California, Georgia, Idaho, Illinois, Maine and Tennessee); but California, Idaho and Maine allowed the physician to use "other usual and customary procedures" and Georgia allowed "other medically recognized criteria" in the determination of death. The definition of brain death in North Carolina requires that, in addition to irreversible cessation of brain function, the person's condition be terminal, incurable and so certified by at least two physicians other than the attending doctor.

Although these operational concepts of death have not been challenged in the courts, attorneys and legal organizations have attempted to formulate a generally acceptable definition of death. Accordingly, several other statements have been proposed by prestigious organizations. The American Bar Association defined death in these terms:

"For all legal purposes, a human body with irreversible cessation of total brain function, according to the usual and customary standards of medical practice, shall be considered dead."

Slightly more specific was the statement drafted by the National Conference of Commissioners on Uniform State Laws:

"For legal and medical purposes, an individual who has sustained cessation of all functioning of the brain, including the brainstem, is dead. A determination of death under this section must be made in accordance with reasonable medical standards."

Burns and Hamlon (79) define death as "the permanent termination of the integrated functioning characteristic of a living body as a whole; in human individuals, beyond the embryonic stage of development, death occurs when there is complete and irreversible loss of functioning of the entire brain."

These statements are open to the criticism that they imply that brain and cardiorespiratory deaths are distinct. Moreover, since medical standards of determining neurological function vary among physicians of different specialities, the operational phrases are imprecise.

A number of states have followed the advice of the House of Delegates

Table IX–1.   The Legal Status of Cerebral Death and Living Wills in the United States of America.

State	Year	Statute (Citation)
Alabama	1979	Cerebral death
Alaska	1974	Cerebral death (Alaska Stats. 09.65.120)
Arizona		None
Arkansas	1979	Cerebral death; Right to die (Ark. 1977, Act 879)
California	1974	Cerebral death (Derring's Cal. Code Ann. Health and Safety, Chap. 3.7, sec. 7180)
		Right to die (Chap. 3.9, sec. 7185)
Colorado		None
Connecticut	1979	Cerebral death
Delaware		None
Florida	1980	Cerebral death (Stats. 382.085)
Georgia	1975	Cerebral death (Code of G. Ann. 88–1715.1)
Hawaii	1978	Cerebral death
Idaho	1977	Cerebral death (Idaho code, 1977, Senate bill No. 1197)
		Right to die (Idaho code, 1977, chap. 45, Title 39)
Illinois	1974	Cerebral death (Smith-Hurd Ill. Ann. Stats. 3, sec 552 B)
Indiana		None
Iowa	1976	Cerebral death (Iowa General Assembly, 1976,
	(1978)	Chap. 1245, sec. 208 and 209)
Kansas	1970	Cerebral death (Kans. Stats. Ann 77–202)
	1977	Natural death (KSA 1976 supp. 65–2837)
Kentucky		None
Louisiana	1976	Cerebral death (Ch. 533, La. Laws of 1976)
Maine	1977	Cerebral death (22MRSA, No. 2846)
		Natural death (22 MRSA, C708) (? passed)
Maryland	1972	Cerebral death (Ann code of Md., art 43, sec 54F)
		Natural death (Ann code of Md., 1977, art. 43, sec. 892–900)
Massachusetts		None
Michigan	1975	Cerebral death (Mich. Pub. Act. 158, Laws of 1975)
Minnesota		None*

*Bills related to cerebral death, right to die or living wills in committee.

of the American Medical Association, which in December, 1974, supported the concept of cerebral death but opposed statutory definitions.

> *Resolved,* That the American Medical Association reaffirm established policy that: "at present, statutory definition of death is neither desirable or necessary"; "that state medical associations urge their respective legislatures to postpone enactment of legislation defining death by statute"; "that death shall be determined by the clinical judgment of the physician using the necessary available and currently accepted criteria"; and "that permanent and irreversible cessation of function of the brain constitutes one of the various criteria which can be used in the medical diagnosis of death." (Substitute Resolution 18).

In Table IX–1, the statutes in the United States of America as of July 1, 1980, regarding cerebral death are listed. Because a number of states have bills related to cerebral death and the right to die in committee, the tabulation may be incomplete. However, the trends toward statutory recognition of cerebral death and the right of an individual to request a dignified demise are apparent; it seems likely that all states will shortly provide legal cognizance of these death concerns (312).

Table IX–1.   The Legal Status of Cerebral Death and Living Wills in the United States of America.

State	Year	Statute (Citation)
Missouri		None
Mississippi		None
Montana	1977	Cerebral death (Mont. HB 0371/02)
Nebraska		None
Nevada	1979	Cerebral death. Right to die (NRS, chap 449, sec 2–16)
New Hampshire		
New Jersey	1976	Cerebral death (1976 Senate No. 992 and 1039)*
		Right to die (Senate No. 1751)
New Mexico	1973	Cerebral death (N. Mex. Stats. Ann., 1–2–2.2)
	1977	Right to die (N. Mex. Laws 1977, chap. 287)
New York		None
North Carolina		Cerebral death (Gen. Stats. Art. 23, No. 90–320)
		Right to die (Gen. Stats. Art. 23, No. 90–322)
North Dakota		None
Ohio		None*
Oklahoma	1975	Cerebral death
Oregon	1975	Cerebral death (Ch. 565, Ore. Laws of 1975)
		Right to die (Senate Bill 434, ch. 183)
Pennsylvania		Cerebral death*
Rhode Island		
South Carolina		None
South Dakota		
Tennessee	1976	Cerebral death* (Pub. Ch. No. 780)
Texas	1979	Cerebral death (Senate bill no. 148)
Utah		None
Vermont		None
Virginia	1973	Cerebral death (Code of Va. sec. 32–364.3:1)
Washington		
West Virginia	1975	Cerebral death (W. Va. Code, sec. 16–19–1(b))
Wisconsin		None
Wyoming	1979	Cerebral death

If an acceptable definition of death could be formulated, many aspects of the determination of the end of life, such as a unified approach, degree of certainty required in usual and unusual cases, etc., could be codified in statutory terms. However, in the present state of uncertain conceptualization, there is grave doubt that this is desirable.

Some attempt has been made to incorporate the criteria for cerebral death into the state laws. In Alabama, such legislation was introduced but failed to get out of committee. In Minnesota, the legalization of brain death criteria was advised as a means of protecting the medical profession which acted on the assumption that cerebral death marked the end of life. However, opposition to this proposal was quite outspoken.

Burns and Hamlon (79) argue that the medical profession is inadequately informed about the medical and legal ramifications of brain death legislation, and so has neither the knowledge nor ability to educate the laity about the principles and significance of cerebral death. Accordingly, to legislate the concept would be premature and might toss a medical responsibility into the political arena.

Tendler (456) points out that physicians and lawyers are loath to draft statutes for the neurological criteria of brain death, lest the definition of death be frozen at a low plane of medical science. The argument that legal recognition of brain death criteria would lessen the likelihood of a physician's being sued for pulling the plug is certainly open to question. Generally speaking, however, there is a concern on the part of physicians that the legal profession might legislate the practice of medicine; if the determination of death were prescribed by law, the precedent could well be carried into other purely medical decisions, to the detriment of the profession. In addition, a statutory set of criteria would infringe upon the judgment of the physician to use other criteria of death.

Mankert (300) presents four arguments against a statutory definition of death:

1. That a law could not cover all aspects of death,
2. That a legal definition would interfere with the patient-doctor relationship,
3. That such a definition would affect the public's attitude towards death,
4. That such a law could lead to a legal recognition and approval of euthanasia.

For these reasons, he asserts that the pronouncement of death should be made on a medical, not a legal, basis.

The conservative respect-for-life groups see brain death legislation as the first step toward legalization of euthanasia. They fear that Judeo-Christian ethics, emphasizing respect for life, would be replaced as the basis for secular policies by humanistic ethics advocating euthanasia, and the right to suicide (79).

The Status of Cerebral Death in the Nations of the World

Although death is pathologically the same in all peoples of the world, its philosophical interpretation varies greatly among the nations, particularly the developing countries. It is thus natural for a new concept of death to be received quite differently in various parts of the world (98,235). On one hand, the technical and medical advances that brought about the brain death concept may not be available in some countries, or, if obtainable, are so only in university centers. In the absence of modern resuscitation procedures, death must be a matter of cessation of cardiac and respiratory function. Hence, in such lands, the populations, even physicians, would have little appreciation of or need for the concept of cerebral death. On the other hand, the major nations of the world, with their elaborate resuscitation equipment, aerate vegetating corpses until cardiac arrest occurs or the physician declares the individual dead on the basis of cerebral death.

From a questionnaire submitted to the Neurosurgical Societies of the world, the current status of cerebral death may be appreciated. With a few exceptions, the concept as a means of proclaiming death of an individual is not legally accepted, even in the major countries of the world (Table IX–2). However, hospital staffs in many countries, operating under rules and regulations that apply specifically to their institution, apply criteria based upon clinical, electrical, rheological and/or biochemical findings.

To appreciate the different national philosophies, the reactions to cerebral death in Europe and South America may be contrasted. In September 1976, at the meeting of the Neurotraumatology Committee of the World Federation of Neurosurgical Societies (held in Brussels), a symposium was held on cerebral death with discussions of the clinical, neuropathological, rheological and metabolic aspects. An attempt was made to formulate criteria of cerebral death that would be acceptable to all participants. However, two views rapidly emerged, the one that the criteria should be based upon clinical considerations with little or no laboratory confirmation, and the other that clinical criteria were inadequate and required electroencephalographic, rheological or metabolic studies to validate the diagnosis of cerebral death. In essence, the proponents of the first view held that with a known diagnosis of an irreparable brain condition, the absence of responsivity, spontaneous respiration and cephalic reflexes for a period of 12 to 48 hours was a simple and satisfactory means of determining the death of a brain that could be used by practically all physicians. The advocates of the second viewpoint held that the diagnosis of cerebral death was particularly applicable to the determination of the death of a prospective organ donor who might suffer cardiac arrest during an observation period of 1–2 days. Moreover, since transplant surgery was only carried out in major, well-equipped hospitals, they considered that sophisticated instrumentation would be available for the establishment of cerebral death in most institutions in which such a diagnosis would be required.

At a workshop sponsored by the Latin American Congresses of Neurosurgery and Electroencephalography, another view regarding cerebral death became apparent. Perhaps influenced by the Napoleonic Code that is the basis of law in most of South America, the representatives of the Latin American countries strongly favored codified legislation on cerebral death. In fact, two of the countries already had passed such laws regarding the determination of cerebral death. Statutory recognition of the concept was considered quite inadequate and, accordingly, a statement was drafted and approved at a plenary session. The text follows:

Table IX–2.   Medical and Legal Status of Cerebral Death.

Country or Region	Concept of Cerebral Death Accepted Medically	Legally	Criteria of Cerebral Death
Argentina	Yes	Yes	Yes
Australia	Yes	Yes	Yes
Austria	Yes	Yes	Yes
Belgium	Yes	No	Yes
Bolivia	Yes	No	Local
Brazil	Yes	No	Local
Canada	Yes	Yes	Yes
Chile	Yes	No	Local
Colombia	Yes	No	Local
Czechoslovakia	Yes	Yes	National
Denmark	No	No	No
Egypt	No	No	No
Finland	Yes	Yes	Yes
France	Yes	Yes	Local
Germany	Yes	No	Yes
Greece	Yes	Yes	Yes
India	No	No	Local
Ireland	Yes	No	Yes
Israel	Yes	No	Local
Italy	Yes	Yes	Yes
Japan	No	No	Local
Korea	Yes	No	Local
Mexico	Yes	Yes	Yes
Netherlands	Yes	No	National
Norway	Yes	Yes	Yes
Pan African	No	No	No
Peru	Yes	No	Local
Poland	Yes	No	Yes
Puerto Rico	Yes	Yes	Yes
South Africa	Yes	No	Local
Spain	Yes	Yes	Local
Sweden	Yes	No	Local
Switzerland	Yes	No	National
Thailand	Yes	No	Yes
Turkey	Yes	No	Local
United Kingdom	Yes	No	National
Uruguay	Yes	No	Local
U.S.A.	Yes	27 States	No
Venezuela	Yes	No	Local
Totals	Yes, 34; No, 5	Yes, 13; No, 25	Local 16 National 19 None 4

Latin American Statement on Cerebral Death.   The XVII Latin American Congress of Neurosurgery and XII Latin American Congress of Electro-Encephalography, at its plenary session June 16th, 1977, reviewed the report of a workshop on cerebral death and approved the following statement.

Advances in medical technology and philosophy have outmoded the concept of death. Accordingly, a revision of the current definition of death is proposed.

Death is the permanent loss of those functions of the brain that are essential to human existence such as the mental and somatic faculties. The loss of such functions may be determined by the traditional methods of ascertaining cardiac arrest which under usual circumstances is followed immediately by loss of cerebral circulation and absence of brain function, or by the usual and customary neurological examinations for brain function. The latter tests are commonly spoken of as criteria for brain death. To aid physicians and surgeons in making this diagnosis, the following proposals provide safe and reliable guidelines for a pronouncement of cerebral death.

In a comatose and mechanically ventilated individual suspected of cerebral death, the diagnosis or cause of the underlying lesion must be established and all appropriate treatment given. When this has been achieved, the enumerated criteria for cerebral death may be applied.

1. Total absence of response to noxiceptive stimulation of the dermatomes supplied by the cranial nerves
2. Absence of spontaneous breathing with complete reliance upon artificial respiration
3. Absence of corneal reflexes
4. Absence of response to vestibular stimulation using 20 cc of ice water for testing each ear
5. Absence of pupillary response to light; the pupils are generally dilated, but if other criteria of CD are met, small or medium sized pupils do not negate the diagnosis
6. Absence of oculocardiac reflex
7. Electrocerebral silence in EEG records made in accordance with the International Federation of Electroencephalography and Clinical Neurophysiology
8. The above findings must be present for a minimum period of 6 hours from their first demonstrations.
9. In the presence of clinical findings of cerebral death, the demonstration, when personnel and equipment are available, that there is no cerebral blood flow or cerebral metabolism for a period of 15 minutes is adequate evidence of a dead brain without further studies.

   Moreover, these criteria or guidelines in exceptional cases of obvious irreparable and lethal brain damage may be abridged and death declared.

It is apparent that the members of the Congresses were willing to accept a broad definition of death that might not be approved by many English-speaking peoples. However, their criteria for cerebral death were more rigid than proposed by many North American and European countries.

The requirement of electrocerebral silence in EEG records made according to the specifications of the International Federation is one that many American and British physicians have deemed not obligatory. As in many other sets of criteria for cerebral death, an option is available for the early pronouncement of death upon rheological or metabolic bases.

The legal criteria of Argentina, Italy and Mexico are similar to American and European standards with few exceptions. The Mexican requirements are similar to those of most North American centers. Some of the criteria have not been founded on scientific data, and collaborative efforts to establish a better basis for their inclusion seems highly desirable since other countries will unquestionably set up requirements based upon these standards. A more precise set of tests could probably be devised that would have equal accuracy.

Argentina

Criteria of Cerebral Death

Law No 21.541. Republica Argentina
Article 21 is amended for the certification of death of a donor who meets the following signs:
1. Total absence of all responses to external stimuli, especially noxiceptive stimuli applied by a needle to the occipital region
2. In non-intoxicated and non-hypothermic patients, a linear EEG record even when sensory or special sensory stimuli are applied, made under the EEG Federation standards for recording cerebral death during 15 minutes and repeated at 6 hours
3. Absence of spontaneous respiration requiring mechanical assistance
4. Dilated or mid-dilated pupils not responding to intense photic stimulation
5. Absence of oculocephalic reflexes
6. Absence of vestibular responses to 200 cc. of ice water
7. Failure of 2–4 mg. of atropine injected intravenously to modify the heart rate in a period of 6 minutes.

Italy

Criteria of Brain Death

National Law of Italy, December 2, 1975, No. 644
1. Deep coma with
   a) muscular atonia,
   b) areflexia of cranial nerves,

c) no plantar reflex,
d) dilated and fixed pupils with absence of corneal responses
2. Absence of spontaneous respiration, even after removal from respirator for 2 minutes
3. No spontaneous or evoked activity in the EEG for 30 minutes on 3 occasions at intervals of 4 hours (a total interval of 12 hours)
4. The clinical findings must be observed and found absent every hour for 12 hours.

Mexico

Criteria of Cerebral Death

Federal regulations for the disposition of organs, tissues, and cadavers of human beings. Diario official, 1976, 338:17–23. Chapter VIII, Article 65.

The methods of determination of the loss of life presented in Article 206 of the Codigo Sanitario de los Estados Unidos Mexicanos are amended by the following criteria:
1. The lack of perception and response to adequate stimuli
2. Absence of the cranial and spinal reflexes
3. Absence of spontaneous respiration
4. Isoelectric electroencephalogram not modified by any stimulus
5. Absence of hypothermia or a history of ingestion of bromides, barbiturates or alcohol.

The above conditions must be present for 24 hours; if cardiac arrest occurs before that time, loss of life is immediately declared.

United Kingdom

Although the statement regarding the diagnosis of brain death by the Conference of Royal Colleges and Faculties of the United Kingdom (399) has no legal sanction, it has been widely accepted and recently sent to all doctors in England and Scotland by the Chief Medical Officers. For this reason, it may be assumed to be the accepted standard for the determination of brain death in the United Kingdom.

Conditions under Which the Diagnosis of Brain Death Should be Considered

1. The patient is deeply comatose.
   a) There should be no suspicion that this state is due to depressant drugs,

b) Primary hypothermia as a cause of coma should have been excluded,
c) Metabolic and endocrine disturbances which can be responsible for or can contribute to coma should have been excluded.
2. The patient is being maintained on a ventilator because spontaneous respiration had previously become inadequate or had ceased altogether. Relaxants (neuromuscular blocking agents) and other drugs should have been excluded as a cause of respiratory inadequacy or failure.
3. There should be no doubt that the patient's condition is due to irremediable structural brain damage. The diagnosis of a disorder which can lead to brain death should have been fully established.

Diagnostic Tests for the Confirmation of Brain Death

All brainstem reflexes are absent:
1. The pupils are fixed in diameter and do not respond to sharp changes in the intensity of incident light,
2. There is no corneal reflex,
3. The vestibulo-ocular reflexes are absent,
4. No motor responses within the cranial nerve distribution can be elicited by adequate stimulation of any somatic area,
5. There is no gag reflex or reflex response to bronchial stimulation by a suction catheter passed down the trachea,
6. No respiratory movements occur when the patient is disconnected from the mechanical ventilator for long enough to ensure that the arterial carbon dioxide tension rises above the threshold for stimulation of respiration,

Other Considerations

1. Repetition of Testing
   It is customary to repeat the tests to ensure that there has been no observer error. This is a matter for medical judgment and repetition time must be related to the signs of improvement, stability, or deterioration which present themselves,
2. Integrity of Spinal Reflexes
   Reflexes of spinal origin may persist or return after an initial absence in brain dead patients,
3. Confirmatory Investigations
   It is now widely accepted that electro-encephalography is not necessary for the diagnosis of brain death.
   Other investigations such as cerebral angiography or cerebral blood-flow measurements are not required for the diagnosis of brain death,

4. Body Temperature

The body temperature in these patients should be not less than 35° C before the diagnostic tests are carried out,

5. Specialist Opinion and The Status of the Doctors Concerned

Decision to withdraw artificial support should be made after all the criteria presented above have been fulfilled and can be made by any one of the following combinations of doctors:

a) A consultant who is in charge of the case and one other doctor,

b) In the absence of a consultant, his deputy, who should have been registered for 5 years or more and who should have had adequate previous experience in the care of such cases, and one other doctor.

The recognition of brain death on the basis of the criteria used by the British medical profession was discussed on the Panarama program of the British Broadcasting Corporation on October 13, 1980.* Admittedly, there are many difficulties in diagnosing a dead brain in the presence of serious heart disease, drug intoxication, and nerve blocking agents. In premature infants, the criteria of cerebral death are poorly established at the present time; many pediatricians hesitate to declare death under such circumstances and rely on the usual somatic signs of cessation of life.

The necessity of ancillary tests such as electroencephalography and angiography which have been required for a diagnosis of brain death in many countries is questioned by British neurologists who rely upon good clinical neurology and asking the right questions. Their search for a clinical syndrome of brainstem death is laudable but they admit that it may have an element of doubt. In view of this uncertainty, which exists to some degree, in practically all sets of criteria of brain death, it would seem advisable to use in every suspected case, several independent parameters to establish the demise of the individual.

---

*Calne, R.Y., Letter to the Editor, The Times, London, October 16, 1980.

Editorial, An Appalling Panorama, Brit Med J, 1980, 281:1028.

Editorial, A television verdict on Brain Death, The Lancet, October 18, 1980.

Johnson, R.W.G., Letter to the Editor, The Times, London, October 16, 1980.

Pallis, C., Medicine and the Media Brit Med J, 1980, 281:1064.

Chapter X

Public Reaction to Cerebral Death

Introduction

The new concept of death as cessation of function of the brain was introduced at a time when the image of the medical profession was somewhat tarnished. The rising cost of medical care (attributed unfairly to fees of gouging physicians), the poorly founded reports of unnecessary surgery and accusations of charges to third-party medical providers for undischarged services, and the impression that doctors were no longer devoted and self-sacrificing but money-grabbing led the general public to regard with suspicion the new means of determining death. This was accentuated when transplant surgeons declared death on this basis in order to obtain organs as soon as possible after death, for the public was not quite sure that enthusiastic surgeons might not be overzealous in their efforts to obtain organs and less critical in the pronouncement of death. Since death ends all, people fear its advent, but dread even more being buried alive.

Premature Pronouncement of Death

From time immemorial, people have been concerned that their death would be prematurely pronounced and that they would be buried alive. In early days this fear was not unfounded, for in the seventh century,

Celsus (92) wrote "furthermore, Democritus, a man of well merited celebrity, has asserted that there are in reality, no characteristics of death sufficiently certain for physicians to rely upon." How frequently the pronouncement of death was premature and how often a cadaver resurrected in a coffin are difficult to determine. The gruesome event occurred sufficiently frequently that Shakespeare wrote of the subject in Romeo and Juliet; Wiertz, a Dutch artist painted a canvas characterizing the situation (see frontispiece); and Count Karnice-Karnicki invented a device that would alert watchers to a resurrection.

In a report on the evacuation of the Fort Randall cemetery, Montgomery (333) describes cadavers "that bore every evidence of having been buried alive." One soldier, struck by lightning, was found in his casket with his legs and arms drawn up as far as possible in the coffin. Another, an alcoholic, was slightly turned, his hands clutching the shrouds. Montgomery states that nearly two percent of those exhumed were victims of suspended animation. Numerous cases were reported in the literature of the nineteenth century. Wilder (512), in a treatise entitled "Burying Alive—A Frequent Peril," cited several persons who were thought to have revived because of the abnormal posture of their limbs when the body was exhumed. More convincing proof was found in the case of a 35-year-old man buried 48 hours after presumed death, whose body was discovered face down with handfuls of hair in his clenched fists and the front and bottom of his coffin shattered. Of course, it must be admitted that other explanations may account for the altered posture of these bodies. Graverobbers, in removing valuables from the interred, not infrequently shifted the cadaver; burrowing animals disturbed the clothing and limbs of their victims; and even the gravediggers, in completing their work, at times broke the often flimsy caskets of the dead.

Judicial courts have recognized the circumstances. In Naples, a woman was buried with all formalities. Some days later, when her grave was reopened to inter another body, the shrouds about the corpse were found torn to shreds, and her limbs broken—apparently in an attempt to free herself. The doctor who had signed the death certificate and the "major" who had authorized interment were tried and each sentenced to three months imprisonment for involuntary manslaughter.

Not a few persons have aroused on the way to their interment, knocked against their coffin and been released. Icard (202) collected a number of cases in which death had been certified by a physician but subsequently the subject had shown signs of life. Although some of these cases only survived a few hours, others enjoyed many years of apparently normal life. Unfortunately, the cause of the suspended animation, whether drugs, alcohol, or systemic illness, is unknown in most of these cases.

The frequency and public fear of premature pronouncements of death have led to the consideration of means to prevent such happenings. In some countries, waiting mortuaries served as a repository for bodies until definite evidence of putrefaction had developed. An attending caretaker or watcher would be warned of the movement of a corpse by the ringing of a bell attached to the cadaver. Extraneous causes agitated the bell much more often than revival of a corpse. These mortuaries were common in Germany in the early part of the nineteenth century.

An ingenious device to alert the outside world if a corpse revived was patented by Count Karnice-Karnicki in Berlin in 1897. This apparatus consisted of a glass ball that rested on the chest of the cadaver and was attached to a tube extending to the outside of the coffin; by means of a series of gears, this device would, upon movement of the chest, admit air and light to the coffin, set a bell ringing and elevate a flag on the tube, so that by one means or another an observer might be alerted to the resurrection (Figure X–1).

Many people in the nineteenth century, alarmed by the prevalence of premature burial, requested, as part of the last offices, that wounds or mutilations be made to assure that they would not awaken. In 1861, Welby (509) recounted how a noble lady instructed that her heart be pierced by a needle, and her body autopsied and embalmed. In fact, embalming received a considerable impetus from the fear of premature burial. Of course, the injection of embalming fluid caused gasps and muscular contractions that the embalmers were assured were not a sign of revival—and would disappear as their work proceeded.

In the last few centuries, the determination of death has been based upon the absence of cardiac and respiratory function. Many novel means have been devised to establish the loss of these vital activities.

To confirm the absence of circulation, a ligature was tied about a finger. If the finger became congested, circulation was present and the individual was considered alive. In 1918, a French law was passed requiring that death should be determined by arteriotomy—if after incision of the temporal or radial artery blood did not flow, death was present. The law further decreed that an intravenous injection of fluorescein should be made. If the individual was alive, the conjunctiva and mucosa of the eye would take on a greenish-yellow coloration within a half hour.

Since arrest of respiration was also a sign of death, various tests were devised to determine if breathing had stopped. For example, a physician would hold a feather in front of the mouth or nose to see if an invisible breath of air would move it, or would put a mirror over the lips of the individual to see if it became dimmed by water vapor of the breath condensing on it. Sometimes a full glass of water was placed on the person's chest; if respiratory movements occurred, the water would spill. In spite of these precautionary measures, an occasional person, particularly if in

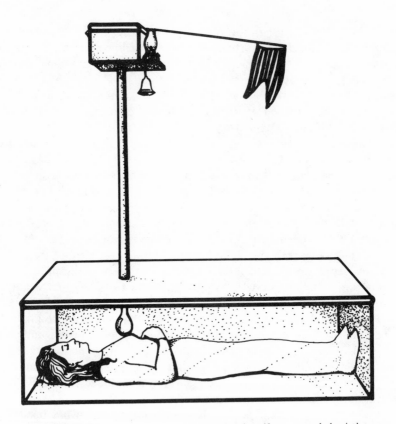

Fig. X–1. A device patented by Count Karnice to assure that, if prematurely buried, a person would make known his or her living state. A glass ball resting on the person's chest was connected to an outside box by a long tube. If the chest moved in respiration, the ball would be displaced, the box above would open to allow air into the coffin, and, by a series of gears, would elevate the flag above the ground and cause the bell to ring. The lamp provided light so that the device could be observed at night.

alcoholic coma or debilitated and exposed to the cold, would be brought into hospitals in a pulseless state, declared dead, but after warming either in the morgue or in a coffin would rise again.

The introduction of cardiac auscultation and later the electrocardiogram made the diagnosis of death relatively errorless, and people lost their fear of premature pronouncement of death.

It was the advent of transplant surgery that revived the public's apprehension that death might be prematurely pronounced and organs removed while life was still extant (335). These fears were fostered by the occasional florid account in the press of persons awakening as incisions were about to be made to remove organs. Such stories were often impossible to verify or deny. However, it is true that improved resuscitative techniques made it possible to revive persons who met the usual criteria of death, namely, absence of perceptible spontaneous respiration and cardiac action. Under conditions of war or major catastrophes, persons in shock have erroneously been diagnosed as dead. In 1967, a soldier who for forty-five minutes had failed to respond to the efforts of a resuscitation team was left for dead, only to be revived by an orderly who detected signs of life as he was about to embalm him (346).

Even in the 1980s, accounts of persons prematurely declared dead and awakening in a morgue may be found in the press (349). These modern Lazaruses usually suffered from hypothermia or drug intoxication, both of which decrease the metabolic requirements to such an extent that abolition or severe depression of cerebral blood flow may be tolerated for an hour. Paramedical personnel and even coroner's physicans are, sometimes, not sufficiently aware of these possibilities.

Reaction to Cerebral Death

The advent of a new concept of determining human death introduced a number of problems. Some related to the means of identifying the morbid state and some to the broader philosophical aspects. The medical problems of certifying cerebral death have been discussed, but implementation of these decisions has created various reactions in both lay and professional circles. Moreover, the considerations regarding restriction of available resuscitative and therapeutic procedures in cases of incurable and irreparable disease were not accepted without serious deliberation in medical, legal, theological and sociological circles.

Reaction of the Medical and Allied Professions

Although most physicians have accepted the concept that death may be based upon the determination of the total and permanent loss of brain function, there have been some opposing viewpoints. These have stemmed both from linguistic differences of opinion and from fundamental conceptual differences. Thus, Byrne et al. (84) argue that inherent in the concept of brain death is the assumption that a specific brain function makes a

person alive. This materialistic concept of human life and its converse—
that cessation of this function represents death—these authors believe is
opposed to the religious beliefs of Christians, Jews, Moslems, Hindus and
other peoples. They argue that the brain has many functions which inte-
grate the actions of different parts of the body. The loss of these functions
does not imply, a priori, the destruction of these parts of the brain, but
only a functional arrest. It is true that this usually leads to destruction and
disintegration of the brain and body, which they consider to be the state
of death; nevertheless, the authors contend that loss of function and destruction are not equivalent. They further argue that irreversible cessation
of function is not the same as destruction of the brain which they equate
with cerebral death.

   This thesis—that it is destruction of the brain, not loss of cerebral function, which is the crucial consideration—is further elaborated. They point
out that irreversible cessation of respiration was long taken as a sure token
of death, but mechanical respirators have invalidated this premise. Not so
long ago the loss of cardiac activity was equated with death, but cardiac
resuscitation has proved this to be incorrect. Even irreversible cessation
of function is unsatisfactory, for the authors imply that what is considered
medically irreversible today may not be tomorrow; something irreversibly
ceasing to function is not destroyed by being permanently idle. Accordingly, they argue that as long as one is dealing solely with irreversible loss
of function, one has a living person; in the case of the brain, as long as
destruction has not occurred, the brain is alive. However, no indication
is given as to how destruction of the brain would be determined. Curran
(112), in a rebuttal of this position, states that "we have traditionally relied
on functional criteria in pronouncing death . . ." not "an anatomic destruction of the heart and lungs." Furthermore, Byrne et al. (84) are not
willing to accept that brain death and personal death are the same. Because
the proponents of brain death will not replace the term "total brain function" by "all brain functions" (the latter includes certain "peripheral"
cerebral activities mediated by a few independently active neurons) Byrne
et al. fear that some characteristic functions of the component parts of the
brain—cortex, brainstem, etc.—may be declared peripheral. Accordingly,
they assert that the Orthodox Jewish position requires "destruction of the
entire brain and only that is . . . an acceptable definition of death." Furthermore, they conclude that the Catholic Church must be as committed
to this concept as Orthodox Jews. However, Protestant theologians are
too widely scattered in their opinions to present a common view.

   From a practical standpoint, Roelofs (397) suggests that the adoption
of irreversible loss of cerebral function as the criterion for total death could
result in violation of an individual's rights, for kidneys could be removed
at a time when, under the cardio-respiratory criteria, the patient would

not be considered dead. Since it is possible to sustain some organs for longer periods of time than others, certain organs would be viable when the patient was declared dead. It is conceivable that cadavers might be sustained indefinitely for research and therapeutic purposes involving certain organs—a macabre prospect. Consequently Roelofs argues that with the new criteria of death, the moral obligations of physicians and society toward the cerebrally dead have to be changed. Furthermore, Roelofs notes that although it might be said that the essence of an individual is his brain, some religions find this objectionable. Religious believers and even the general laity look upon the body as a machine or a house operated by the soul. According to this belief, the body is essential to eating, drinking, dancing, singing, making love and other aspects of human living, and to assume that the brain alone is the essential organ is incorrect. Given this point of view, it is easy to see why not all people could accept the concept of cerebral death.

Although physicians, lawyers and theologians generally accepted the concept of cerebral death, there remained a number of problems that were not readily resolved. Most of these concerned the actions necessary for the proper disposition of the beating heart corpse. The first questions related to the pronouncement of death.

Time of Death.   In the traditional methods of pronouncing death, the failure of the person's vital functions herald the moment of death, but in brain death there is no such obvious point. Accordingly, arbitrary standards have been set up as guides. The time of death is defined as that time when the person first met the criteria for cessation of brain function; however, the declaration of death is made when the patient has been observed long enough to establish the irreversibility of the state. This arbitrary dichotomy could conceivably cause legal difficulties.

Pronouncement of Death.   The law has given physicians the responsibility for determining death, but with the ever-present threat of malpractice suits, medical institutions and doctors are loath to make any declaration that may be contested. Hence, some hospitals require the consent of relatives before discontinuing treatment of a brain-dead patient. However, this seems inappropriate, for relatives are certainly not in a position to decide whether or not a person is dead. A further difficulty arises when organ donation is contemplated, for a possible conflict of interest may well arise. To avoid such possible complications, most hospitals have set up their own standards for the determination of cerebral death and the related protocol. The Harvard criteria suggested that the attending physician, after consultation with other doctors involved in the case, should pronounce death. However, later criteria have suggested that a consultant, unassociated with the case, should give the second opinion so that is is independent and unbiased by previous professional relations or personal interests in the donee. Even then, many attending physicians dislike acknowledging death, and leave the distasteful task of entering orders to discontinue all therapy to the nurse, who understandably resents this imposition and potential liability.

Institutional Regulation of Encephalothanasia.   To assure that the criteria of cerebral death were adequately met, many hospitals in the U.S.A. appointed brain death committees, usually composed of an internist, a neurologist or neurosurgeon, and an electroencephalographer, whose duty was to review the history and examine the patient before any case suspected of cerebral death had resuscitative efforts abandoned. This committee acted as consultants to the attending physician and advised the latter of their opinion regarding the presence of a dead brain. The physician made the pronouncement of death, after which all resuscitative measures were stopped and the corpse given the usual services. If organ transplant was being considered, it was thought essential that none of the consultants on the cerebral death committee have any relationship to the treating physicians or to the transplant surgeons. Under such circumstances, if permission for organ removal had been obtained, the declaration of death was made in the operating room after the patient had been surgically prepared. In the occasional case pronounced cerebrally dead on the ward, efforts to maintain the systemic circulation in order to perfuse the donor organs have been misinterpreted by nursing and paramedical personnel, and have caused emotional reactions.

As cerebral death became commonplace, the rigorous criteria and requirement of verification by a committee were relaxed. However, a consultation by an independent senior physician was required before the attending physician could declare a patient cerebrally dead. The criteria to be used were formulated in accord with the generally accepted national standards in consideration of the facilities available in the institution. Accordingly, some hospitals followed clinical criteria that had to be present for some days, while others, after a short period of observation, verified death by electrocerebral silence or absence of cerebral blood flow.

Relationship to the Medical Examiner.   The use of cerebral death as a determinant of death does not change a physician's relationship with the medical examiner or coroner. If suspicion of a traumatic origin and the possibility of criminal liability exists, the office of the medical examiner must be notified; if the cause of death is not clear or suspicion of foul play is entertained, similar notification is mandatory.

The reference to the medical examiner becomes more consequential when organ removal is contemplated, especially if death is possibly due to criminal assault. The medical examiner has a duty to examine the body to determine the cause of death and positively identify criminal violence. This requirement may interfere with organ removal, for the medical examiner must have the entire body for his inspection and certification; accordingly, his release of the body is essential before an organ can be removed. Usually, the physician obtains a telephonic release of the body at or about the time of death, so that the organs may be taken out under ideal conditions, and the medical examiner can complete his study at his convenience. However, cases have occurred in which the medical examiner would not release the body, and although permission had been obtained for organ removal and postmortem examination, these procedures could not be done. Such difficulties usually arise only when the cause of death is criminal assault, and the assailant is being held on a charge of murder. Under these circumstances, it is wise to omit organ removal so that the medico-legal picture is not confused by two possible causes of death. Moreover, as noted previously, the transplant surgeon may be accused of murder should any question arise that the victim's death was not due to the primary disorder. This point arose in a Houston case in which the healthy heart of a gunshot victim was being considered for transplant. However, the definition of death was the traditional heart-lung function. After the medical examiner was notified and found the victim with a good heartbeat, the transplant surgeons, in the absence of the medical examiner, declared the patient dead and removed the heart. The defense for the person accused of the shooting was that the victim's death was not the result of the gunshot wound but the surgeon's actions, especially as the medical examiner had found the victim alive just a few minutes before the removal of the heart. The case was settled by the defendant's case bargaining (498).

The Transplant Surgeon and Cerebral Death.   The advent of transplant surgery gave an impetus to the formulation of a practical concept of death that did not rely upon the cessation of systemic circulation. This gained importance as surgeons realized that an organ removed for transplantation some time after cardiac arrest is often poorly accepted by a recipient. Although the early enthusiasm for cardiac transplants was dampened by the high mortality, a more conservative approach has engendered an optimistic outlook for selected patients. In a recent review of seven years' experience, Schroeder et al. (416) state that human cardiac transplants prolong human life of otherwise healthy young individuals. If the individual survives the first 3 months, there is a 75% survival at the end of one year and a graded improvement thereafter. The greatest problem remains the acute or chronic rejection of the allograft. The early diagnosis of rejection is aided by serial percutaneous transventricular endomyal cardiac biopsies of the right ventricle. Of the survivors, 88% are vocationally rehabilitated; however, some suffer from the complications of immunosuppressor therapy.

Renal transplantaton, which had a slower and less spectacular beginning, has had an even better record. In the beginning, kidney transplants were taken from living relatives or volunteers, but as the technique became standardized and the demand greater, the source of grafts shifted. In 1975, renal transplants were taken from cadavers in 53% of cases in the U.S.A., in 79% in Europe, and in 98% in Australia. With the increase in the number of possible recipients, the availability of donor organs, in spite of collaborative programs for utilization, has become a problem. This is due in part to the high attrition rate, for only approximately 25% of potential donor organs are eventually used. In a recent paper, Chatterjee et al. (94) stated that of 86 organs referred for possible transplantation only 22 were actually used. This may seem an extreme example, and, indeed, Flatmark's figures are somewhat better. He reported that of 69 potential donors 26 were not used (136). Thus, although analyses from morbidity statistics may indicate an adequate source of donor organs, in practice the supply is insufficient to meet the needs. In 1973, of 642 recipients waiting for kidney transplants only 175 received cadaver organs.

Since, at the present time, transplant surgeons are loath to use organs, particularly kidneys, from other than beating-heart cadavers, the pronouncement of death must be on the basis of brain death. This poses both technical and ethical problems.

The ideal cases for donor organs are rarely patients with chronic incurable afflictions. Too often these individuals have systemic disease affecting the organs that might be transplanted. Young persons with acute traumatic or vascular lesions of the brain are more appropriate donors. However, the certification of cerebral death in these individuals poses a problem since their cerebral lesions are often rapidly lethal. Hence, it may be impossible for such cases to meet the commonly accepted criteria of cerebral death before their heart arrests. Consequently, these donors may have to be declared dead on other criteria than cerebral death. But this introduces legal problems that can only be avoided if the near relatives are altruistic enough to grant permission for removal of organs from the moribund person. To meet legal requirements after informed consent has been obtained from the next of kin, these patients may be taken to the operating room and surgically prepared for the removal of donor organs. When cardiac arrest occurs, the patient is certified dead, and the organs may then be removed from the cadaver.

If time is not so critical and the victim's cardiovascular state is satisfactory, the transplant team can wait until the criteria of cerebral death are met and then remove the organs from a beating-heart cadaver. Such organs are considered to have a somewhat better chance of being received and functioning in the recipient. For this purpose, criteria of cerebral death confirmed by a test indicating the absence of cerebral blood flow seem particularly desirable. On this basis, the diagnosis may be established within a few hours of the primary insult.

However, the rights of the moribund person must be carefully guarded lest, in the enthusiasm to restore life to an ailing donee, they be infringed upon. There is no legal basis to neglect or even abridge the rights of the dying in order to bring health to a young teenager in need of an organ. Accordingly, the death protocol must provide safeguards not only for the patient but for the physician who otherwise may be suspect of being less critical in the determination of death when organs are to be removed for transplantation. It is particularly important that the most up-to-date and precise assessment of the dying patient's state be made, even if this means that organs must be sacrificed because the techniques for an absolute diagnosis of death are not available.

Another consideration in the evaluation of a person *in extremis* is that the patient be exposed to as little risk as possible in carrying out diagnostic procedures to determine death. Even minor stresses may prove too much for the person hovering between life and death. For these reasons a rigid adherence to the hospital protocol is essential.

Reaction of Nurses and Paramedical Personnel. The concept of cerebral death has drawn reactions from all individuals involved in the care of the patient. Since the consequences of such a declaration—the removal of mechanical aids assisting vital functions—are so different from the usual principles of health care, nurses and even some doctors regard them as a violation of the Hippocratic oath. It is not surprising, then, that consultant "brain death teams" seeing a patient to determine cerebral death are looked upon with the abhorrence and aversion accorded vultures. On some occasions, these feelings have been so acute that technicians have refused to work on the team, for paramedical and even medical personnel look upon these procedures as contrary to the previous therapeutic goals.

This feeling has engendered a revulsion on the part of some nursing personnel toward the performance of their postmortem duties. The "pulling of the plug" and removal of intratracheal and nasogastric tubes are distasteful tasks, even after the person has been declared cerebrally dead. At times, physicians make these attentions even more difficult by neglecting to write "death orders."

Creighton (107) has emphasized the troubles that nurses encounter in getting doctors to assume their legal responsibilities. "When faced by the problem and the refusal of the physician to come and examine the patient, the nurse should chart the time and the signs and symptoms and the actions taken." Verbal orders at such times are certainly undesirable, and if accepted, should be countersigned as soon as possible. Creighton states that nurses should consider the legal implications—which may endanger their future—if they take on extraneous, improperly delegated medical tasks.

The psychological situation becomes even more stressful when, after a decision of brain death has been made, transplant surgeons take over the care of the patient. In order to improve the state of the organs to be removed, they may order more fluids and vasopressor agents, thus creating a paradoxical condition for the nursing service who would ordinarily be preparing the corpse for removal from the clinical unit. This has caused serious emotional conflicts that may be avoided if the total health team is adequately instructed in the necessities for organ removal. If the nursing corps understands the total program of dying and transplantation, their cooperation can be readily obtained and the paradox mentioned above will either not arise or will be viewed in proper perspective.

The nurse also frequently encounters problems unrelated to her personal or professional feeling for the patient, for she is often the one who must inform and console the grieving family. This requires not only an empathic but a sympathetic and often emotional effort on the nurse's part. In discussing the management of the relatives of a brain death patient, Butcher (83) notes that strains above and beyond those usually associated with a death are encountered, for frequently the shocked family members have had no time to prepare themselves emotionally and mentally for the crisis. Hence, the nurse must not only carry out her medical duties but assume certain intimate responsibilities in order to help the family adjust to the realities and to alleviate their grief and apprehensions. This may involve attention to special social and religious customs demanded by the patient's culture. This type of assistance is often shared with the clergy to the advantage of both.

Special problems may be encountered when nursing personnel from countries with concepts of death quite foreign to those of the United States of America are attending the dying. To indoctrinate these persons, religious mentors of their native lands may discuss the current theological reactions to cerebral death.

Theological Considerations

Brain Death and Theology.   The question has been raised whether the concept of cerebral death is compatible with theological views of death. Obviously, theological concepts of death vary with the religious denomination. Judaism, Protestantism and Roman Catholicism, to mention the three most populous religious groups in the United States, have different views on life and death.

The Orthodox Jewish law recognized many indices of life and death. Throughout Rabbinical literature the essence of life is respiration. In the story of creation, God "breathed life" into the nostrils of man. Consequently, breathing in traditional Jewish theology is more important than the beating of the heart. The Code of Laws was well aware of a state resembling cerebral death, for beheading was a common experience. The agonal throes of a decapitated man were looked upon as the aftermath of death, and not as evidence of life. Thus, cerebral death is readily understood as a physiological state analogous to decapitation; respiration, a critical criterion of life, is lost as well as the higher integrative functions, so the pronunciation of death may be made on Biblical standards. The fact that heart action persists is not consequential, since its cessation is considered a cause, not evidence, of death.

Roman Catholic theologians have based the moment of death upon the time of departure of the soul from the body. Although the latter is not an objectively measurable event, the signs of apparent death—apnea and asystole—have been accepted as reasonably accurate indicators of the moment of real death. It has been reasoned that Roman Catholic theologians would be even more willing to accept irreversible cessation of brain function as an indication of the departure of the soul and hence the moment of death (479).

Protestant theologians have taken no consistent stand on the brain death issues, but outstanding writers have accepted the concept of brain-related criteria for the pronouncement of death (479).

Thus, the major religious bodies in the USA have found no difficulty in integrating the new concept of death into the teachings of their churches.

Theological View of Death. Although death is commonly considered to have an awful face, it must be admitted that death should not always be considered malevolent; it can be quite benevolent. Consider the sentiment of Old Man River—"tired of living, feared of dying"—and the thousands of pain-wracked persons who looked upon death as a salvation. Certainly death, in itself, is not necessarily evil, and to fight it may be quite unethical or even immoral.

Yet Jewish law decrees that the physician has an obligation "to use every ability within his power to save the lives of his fellow men." Even today some physicians maintain "that he (the physician) must carry on until the issue is taken out of his hands." But the problem becomes more difficult by reason of the scientific advances that make it possible to maintain life functions mechanically, at least, for some periods of time. How obligated is the physician to use these elaborate and expensive methods of resuscitation? Pope Pius XII answered this question in these words:

"It is incumbent on the physician to take all reasonable, ordinary means of restoring the spontaneous vital functions and consciousness, and to employ such extraordinary means as are available to him to this end. It is not obligatory, however, to continue to use extraordinary means indefinitely in hopeless cases"(379).

One might ask, what constitutes "extraordinary means"? Healley (89) defines this term as being "whatever . . . is very costly or very unusual, or very painful, or very difficult, or very dangerous, or if the good effects that can be expected from its use are not proportionate to the difficulties and inconveniences that are entailed." In another vein, Archbishop Lambruschini (89) explained that "If the prolonging of life is uncertain or if one can expect hardships, pain and the need for costly and continued treatment, remedies may be considered extraordinary and not binding on the consciences of patients' relatives and doctors."

Obviously, the term defies precise definition and leaves much to the judgment and philosophical background of the attending physician.

Thus, it seems that the papal annunciation implies that "extraordinary means" cannot be withheld if they are at hand, but may be discontinued if the outlook becomes hopeless. In common language, there is an obligation to put in the plug in the first place, and this inherently introduces the question of the right and/or obligation to pull out the plug. The Church sidesteps this issued by asserting that it is a medical, not a theological decision, although it is commonly referred to as a question of who wi play God.

Rabbi Segal (423) states this explicity: "If something artificial is inhibiting the normal process of dying, as for example, if a respirator is used to keep the patient alive, or injections are being used on the patient in order to prolong his 'life,' the inhibitor may be removed and the person allowed to die."

Certain fundamentalist groups hold inflexible tenets regarding the moment of death that permit no concepts contrary to Biblical teaching to be incorporated in medical or legal definitions. They fear that even well-intentioned men in a highly esteemed profession may transgress the bounds of moral or ethical law in the determination of the moment of death when colleagues are pressuring to obtain organs for transplanting as early as possible. The public is aware of these influences and fearful that physicians may yield to them on the excuse that the end justifies the means. If physicians take the public into their confidence and fully inform them of the problems, the people will be willing advocates of an early determination of the moment of death.

Theology and Organ Transplantation.   When organs are to be removed for transplant, many other theological problems arise. Although today Catholic theology finds no fault in the use of tissues or organs of animals or man for implantation into the body of a human being, it must be remembered that only 300 years ago a heteroplastic cranioplasty had to be taken down upon threat of excommunication, because it was decreed that the bone of a dog was not befitting the head of a Christian gentleman (315). However, religion is not static, but keeps up with the advances of science, so that "Rabbinical authorities agreed that the transplant of the heart of Denise Darvall, an Anglican Christian girl, into the body of Louis Washkansky, a Jewish businessman, did not transgress the laws of the Jewish religion."

Many other theological aspects are encountered in organ transplantation—the right and obligation to donate organs, the rights of the recipients, the ethics of performing transplant surgery and the selection of recipients, especially if donor organs must be rationed. However, these questions are beyond the bounds of this treatise.

Chapter XI

Broad Implications

Introduction

In this treatise, a careful distinction has been made between death of a brain, and irreversible coma and irreparable brain damage. The latter subjects are perhaps equally pertinent in the eyes of the general public, for although brain death will require only a short period of hospitalization after which cardiac arrest will occur, these other conditions often need long periods of intensive care in hospital or home, sometimes with little chance of a fatal outcome for years. Accordingly, although the individual may have none of the qualities which commonly are ascribed to human life—such as communication, motility, emotions, personality—he or she may continue a vegetative existence. Whether or not such individuals should be maintained in this state for indefinite periods is a serious ethical and moral consideration not only to relatives, but to physicians and sociologists as well.

Two main kinds of chronic brain impairment produce such states. The one is the irreversible coma, which may be the result of an injury to the brain, an infection of the brain or a side effect of a respiratory or cardiac failure in which resuscitation was not achieved quickly enough. Perhaps the best known example of this is the Quinlan case, which received extensive media coverage. This comatose and unresponsive girl, who had some cranial nerve reflexes, feeble respiratory efforts and an active electroencephalogram, at no time met the criteria for cerebral death. Accordingly, the physicians refused to discontinue resuscitative efforts (400). The father was appointed by the Court as the girl's guardian with authority to "pull the plug" if the family agreed to that decision, the attending physician averred that there was no reasonable chance of recovery, and the ethics committee of the hospital concurred in this prognosis. Under these circumstances the Court ruled that there would be no liability. However, when respiratory assistance was discontinued, the girl maintained spontaneous respiration but remained in a comatose and unresponsive condition. In such circumstances, the unresponsive individual does not have a complete and total cessation of function of the brain, but certain brainstem centers which might be considered vital are still functioning. Thus, such an individual may breathe, maintain a good circulation, and if fed by stomach tube or some other means live almost indefinitely.

The second impairment relates to an individual who has some limited contact with the environment, albeit only by eye movements. The latter condition, which has been termed the "locked-in-syndrome," results from damage to the upper brainstem, causing a paralysis of all four extremities while leaving intact the lower part of the brainstem; thus, respiration is possible, blood pressure may be maintained, and the individual, receiving stimuli from the spinal cord and cerebral cortex, may perceive the environment and respond by movement of the eyes.

Responsibility to Initiate Resuscitation.   The question then arises as to the moral responsibility of physicians and families to maintain such individuals by extraordinary means when it is obvious that they never will be able to participate in social activities nor to have the interpersonal relationships which characterize a normal individual. What is the responsibility of the physician to these individuals? The current law does not give a clear answer. Certainly, the physician may give a medical opinion as to the value of treatment in maintaining and restoring a patient's life; the judgment need only be one which reasonable doctors of similar training and experience might reach. The final decision regarding the physician's recommendations is up to the patient, if he or she is competent; it is not clear whether the next of kin can make such decisions. This indefinite situation is further confused by the uncertainty as to whether failure to initiate treatment will be construed as only a passive neglect or as an active agent precipitating death. Oden (353) believes that under two circumstances— the permanent loss of cognitive functions and the irrefutable evidence of imminent death—one may omit extraordinary treatment with the consent of the patient or next of kin. Certainly if, at the time of an insult—cardiac, cerebral or other—it is possible to determine that the damage is irreparable, many physicians would decide (pending the approval of the next of kin) not to apply extraordinary resuscitative medical measures that would subject the individual to an interminable coma, which might deplete the family emotionally and financially (478). This judicious neglect is rarely considered for professional or criminal sanctions. At the same time, any lack of unanimity or a dissenting opinion of any medical consultant would necessitate intensive care, for a controversy might take the case before ethics committees, or even the courts.

Of course, a physician's judgments might be modified by other factors, such as age, life expectancy, religious beliefs, etc. This is not to suggest leaving NTBR (not to be resuscitated) orders on every patient over 65 years of age, irrespective of his or her medical history and provisional diagnosis. That would seem both unethical and immoral. Perhaps most of the aged with cardiac arrest do succumb before their ribs, fractured during resuscitation, have healed. Still, establishing an arbitrary age limit for resuscitation is inhumane. Yet, for the physician, trained to do everything possible to save life, to withhold extraordinary therapies requires much soul searching. The physician has only a few guidelines available to help in this sort of dilemma. When less than 3 minutes have elapsed since cardiac or respiratory arrest occurred, and if the primary condition is not a lethal but a reversible state (such as drowning, electric shock, etc.), the physician should spare no effort. Children and infants often have complete recovery after 4 or even 6 minutes of cardiac arrest. Newborns, especially premature neonates, may survive quite long periods of anoxia.

The role of the patient, parents or guardians in such decisions is not entirely clear. On rare occasions, the patient may be sufficiently alert to express an opinion regarding the use of extraordinary means to prolong life. Usually the next of kin must have the circumstances explained so that their informed consent be obtained. Even with that approval, the decision to withhold unusual therapies is a delicate and difficult judgment on the part of the attending physician, who must act contrary to his long training.

If cardiac arrest occurs in situations where a layman trained in first aid is available to initiate and carry out resuscitation, he or she is duty bound to attempt resuscitation of every case of cardiac standstill and to maintain the effort until a physician arrives. Under these circumstances, the doctor is bound to continue the activity and to make a judgment as to its probable outcome. In the favorable case, respiration will resume shortly after thoracic massage has been started; such a train of events indicates that the anoxic period was not long and that complete cerebral restitution may be expected. The later the return of respiration, the worse the prognosis. When no more effective means than mouth-to-mouth resuscitation and external cardiac massage are available, full recovery very seldom ensues if there is no response within 15 minutes, and after 30 minutes the chances of survival are practically nil.

If there are means for defibrillation, internal massage, artificial ventilation and the control of acidosis, the prognosis is better. The patient's response may be evaluated by checking the respiration, cardiac action and, if possible, the electroencephalogram. As long as these functions seem to be improving, the physician should be encouraged that the efforts may save the patient. The eventual outcome will depend upon the severity of the injury suffered by the patient before and during the procedure of revival as well as the doctor's skill in resuscitation. Since the aim is not to prolong dying, nor to create cripples, nor to maintain breathing corpses, all efforts may be abandoned after a reasonable period of time if cardiac and cerebral functions show no signs of returning.

Responsibility to Discontinue Resuscitation

An even more critical question, and one quite germane to the topic of brain death, concerns the discontinuance of extraordinary measures once they have been initiated. Relatives of patients frequently confuse the issue of whether a person is dead with whether the patient should be allowed to die. This is particularly true when mechanical means are being used for pulmonary ventilation. Lay people assume that such ventilation is adequate for life support and that its removal would allow the patient to die. It takes a considerable understanding for the laity to realize that the necessity for such measures often is an indication that the individual is already dead, and that only a beating-heart cadaver is being artifically respirated.

Yet medical ethics dictate that the physician, in all but a few exceptional cases, use all the modern facilities available to maintain life. And once initiated, both medical and legal tradition require that a patient be treated in a reasonable manner "as long as the case requires" (89). Irrespective of a merciful intent to relieve pain and suffering, deliberate nonfeasance to cause death is considered punishable homicide. Thus, the withdrawal of life-support systems is potentially subject to charges of homicide. Because the patient is helpless and unable to express his wishes, the courts have held that once a life-support system has been started, there is a moral and legal obligation to continue its use as long as it is maintaining life. Of course, when life has ceased as determined by cardiorespiratory or cerebral criteria, there is no longer any need to persist in treatment, but death should be declared before the plug is pulled. However, as long as life is extant, the discontinuance of life-support systems should only be carried out by order of a court of law. In this way, the physician is relieved of a decision which is often abhorrent.

Occasionally a condition arises in which the patient should be continued on a respirator with vasopressor drugs after it seems certain that the brain is dead. Such an example is the case of a female in the late stage of pregnancy whose maintenance may provide time for a viable baby to be delivered, or a patient with a hopeless condition for whom mechanical support may allow viable organs to be removed for transplant. However, the physician must make these decisions, usually after consultation with other physicians or specialists in resuscitation. If organs are being considered for transplant, it is prudent to have as a consultant someone entirely unrelated to either the previous care of the patient or the transplant team.

The Right to Die a Natural Death

These considerations logically lead to the question of the right to die, which has troubled thinking people since scientific advances eliminated mortality but left an even more fearful and awesome morbidity. Now that the "friend of the aged" has been almost conquered, the aged all too frequently decay and rot in nursing homes and hospitals that must provide the best and most modern care, when all the patient wants or needs is to be allowed a short and not too painful demise. This topic has been the subject of many essays in lay publications and of editorials in medical journals. The publicity associated with the Quinlan case has accentuated the concern, stimulating a rash of bills in legislatures throughout the country to provide the terminally ill patient with the legal right to a dignified demise. The California legislature was the first to pass such a bill, but many other states have followed (Table IX–1). Perhaps these formal statements will allay fears of the elderly that they will be given technical therapy that will only extend a vegetative existence and exhaust their savings. Since life ultimately has a fatal outcome, some consideration should be given to making the inevitable as salutary as modern science can.

To this end, a "Living Will" has been proposed as a means of assuring a graceful termination of life. Composed and signed by the individual at a time when he or she is mentally competent, the Living Will reads: "If in the course of a terminal illness from which there is no reasonable expectation of recovery from physical disability in the opinion of two physicians, I request that I be allowed to die and not to be kept alive by artificial means or heroic measures." It is to be implemented when the individual is incapable of speaking for him- or herself—in most cases, when the individual is unconscious. These wills are legally binding in some dozen states. Moreover, a companion bill, introduced in several states, protects doctors and hospitals who follow these instructions from malpractice suits for not employing extraordinary means to maintain life.

A few opponents of this law regard it as a means of legalizing "mercy killings." Some consider it a usurpation of God's power, quoting "there is a time to be born and a time to die" (Ecclesiastes III). Others oppose the proposal on the grounds that the dying process is not an appropriate subject for legislation. While recognizing that the California Natural Death Act upheld the principle that there was no obligation to continue unusual treatment when death is imminent, Capron and Kass (87) considered that its wording confused rather than clarified the law. However, most people who have expressed an opinion, particularly doctors, nurses and paramedical personnel, favor this means of providing patients a legal right to express their wishes regarding their demise.

Borderline Problems

Borderline problems of life and death are discussed only to present cerebral death in a proper perspective, for without such a background the inherent issues in and responsibilities for controlling the process of passing from life to death may be quite confusing.

The situation is particularly sensitive when the patient is young, and perhaps the only child of his parents. Under these circumstances, there is the desire to maintain life as long as possible. Certainly, the parents are entitled to have the best health measures for their infant, even though it means caring for a vegetating individual indefinitely, for children have survived in a vegetating state for more than 10 years. Provided the family is not in straitened financial circumstances, there seems no moral or ethical reason why medical measures should be withheld. However, relatively few families have either the philosophical mind or the financial facilities to provide such care. Without doubt, the presence of a vegetating child or adult creates a mental and physical stress on a family, for parents usually feel that it is their duty to provide personal services to the vegetating offspring, but in so doing they may deprive other more fortunate members of the family of their just attention and love.

The problem becomes more acute when third parties are responsible for the care of such individuals. If the parents or relatives do not have to provide the financial backing for medical care, they are apt to be demanding of third parties who have a certain responsibility; yet, the question might well be raised as to whether there is a legal or ethical responsibility to maintain an individual in a vegetative state indefinitely. Courts of law have indicated that it would be illegal to do anything which would shorten or abruptly cause the termination of life. On the other hand, there are many extraordinary measures which might not be introduced and maintained. Certainly, in religious circles, this problem has been recognized, and the Pope has indicated that there comes a time in the care of a vegetating individual when extraordinary measures for health care need not be continued, and their withdrawal or omission should not be considered a moral dereliction (379).

This is an area in which legislation is badly needed at the present time. The medical profession has recognized the problem, and yet has not been able to resolve it satisfactorily. The issue may be settled quietly in individual cases, but in general it constitutes a serious decision. The methods by which this may be resolved, theoretically, are numerous, but in practice are somewhat limited. This is related to the problem of euthanasia, where an individual, quite competent, may desire that his suffering and life be terminated. However, the law does not recognize the right of the individual nor of his attendants to hasten or induce death. Accordingly, it has been suggested that a committee of medical consultants, sociologists, theologians and legal representatives might review a case of an individual who has been hibernating and obviously has no chance of recovery to a normal state. If this reviewing body determined that normal life was impossible and that extraordinary means required to maintain life were constituting financial difficulties or depleting the resources of a family or even transferring from normal individuals of a family to a vegetating member the love and affection which should be given the normal persons, then that committee could recommend that medical measures to maintain life be discontinued. This need not require that life be terminated by physical or pharmacological means, but simply that the extraordinary means of maintaining life no longer be continued.

Other methods of meeting this problem have been suggested: some have consisted of simply a frank discussion between the family and the guardians of the individual and the physician. Under such circumstances, the physician might be willing to discontinue most of the extraordinary means of maintaining life, or the family, who in some cases are responsible for the care of the individual, might unconsciously become less meticulous in their care of the individual, so that bedsores, pneumonia and/or infections might quickly terminate the issue. In not a few instances, members of the family have taken it upon themselves to remove tubes and stop feedings when they have concluded that the outlook for their beloved was completely hopeless. In a few cases, they have persuaded nurses or other paramedical personnel to administer pharmacological agents which would terminate cardiac activity. However, in many cases the issue has been settled without going to this length by simply being less active in the care of the individual (308).

Another aspect of this problem relates to the care of a newborn baby who enters the world with serious neurological defects. An anencephaly, severe meningomyelocele, or teratology involving intestines and heart may make it difficult or impossible for such children to survive more than a few weeks. The question arises under such circumstances as to the moral obligation of the parent, the physicians, and society. What effort should be made to salvage such babies, who, it is obvious, will not be able to reach even childhood? Here, again, the question has been variously answered in the past. Unquestionably, many obstetricians and pediatricians, involved in the delivery of a very seriously defective child whom they know will not be able to survive indefinitely, have decided to omit the extraordinary methods of resuscitation and to withhold any therapy which might prolong life. In some cases, physicians do not even attempt to resuscitate such children, and simply report to the parents that the child was dead at birth. However, sometimes the parents are extremely emotionally attached to the defective child, especially if it happens to be the first-born, and are insistent upon everything possible being done, even though they are told that the child cannot live for more than a few weeks.

There are, of course, many congenital abnormalities which are not completely incompatible with life for some period of time, and the question then arises as to whether it is desirable to maintain a functioning brain and organs which, it is admitted, will never develop into a sapient human being. These problems are extremely difficult to resolve, and the response of physicians varies considerably. There is in the minds of most physicians the thought that they should do everything posible to save a human being who has some potential for a conscious existence. Others pay more attention to the quality of that existence; consequently, they consider that it would not be moral to continue the technical maintenance of a severely defective newborn, if that individual would not at some future time be able to maintain life independently, free of pain and suffering. The question becomes even more difficult when it seems that survival would mean a lifetime of institutional care or repeated medical crises demanding frequent hospital admissions and operations. These issues are particularly traumatic to the mothers who have gone through a trying pregnancy in anticipation of a normal child. Consequently, a great deal of consideration must be given by the physicians, relatives and parents to the decision whether or not to sustain an infant's life. If a child's life is saved, it may be even more traumatizing to the parents, particularly to the mother, when she sees the deformity and eventually realizes the hopelessness of the total situation.

The problem is not one which is entirely within the prerogative of the physician. Not infrequently, a court order may be required to discontinue treatment of a seriously deformed child, particularly if there is a difference of opinion between parents and attending physicians. Some parents who have several children may refuse permission for a surgeon to treat a defective child who might, with extraordinary surgical measures, live for an undefinite period of time. Accordingly, in some cases, it is necessary for the court to appoint a guardian in order to have surgical procedures carried out. Moreover, there is the likelihood in such cases, where the child's life is spared initially, that the parents will take little care of it, so that its chances of indefinite survival in a deformed state would be very slight. In some cases, when the total picture seemed hopeless, physicians have allowed an infant with severe congenital abnormalities to die from malnutrition, even though it might have been possible to correct an alimentary defect. These broad problems are arbitrarily settled at the present time by decisions more related to the psychological and financial state of the parents than to ethical and moral standards or social approbation.

At some time in the future, these basic questions about the prolongation of life in babies with incurable defects must be resolved. Is it necessary that the physician do all possible for newborns, or only the usual and customary measures? What guidelines should the physician have in recommending treatment and advising parents? Obviously, the parents should have the final decision as to what unusual and extraordinary therapeutic procedures should be carried out. Yet their viewpoint may be warped by their social and financial status. Accordingly, when it seems that moral injustice is being done, legal process may be necessary to obtain guardians for such children. These problems, which are peripheral to the question of cerebral death, nevertheless require consideration in medical circles, in legal organizations, and in society. They are problems which, with the increasing availability of resuscitative measures, are becoming more acute; in fact, it may well be that, if all individuals born with defects are treated, then the unfit will survive, whereas the healthy may not be able to use all of the facilities which would otherwise be available.

Perhaps another aspect related to this question is the consideration of whether or not fetuses with hereditary diseases that are diagnosed in utero should be aborted. In general, such has been the case, but there may well be instances in which interruption of these pregnancies would be undesirable. Here, again, the social, financial and physical state of the mother and father, as well as other considerations not entirely medical, are of paramount importance.

These questions, which are on the periphery of the general problem of cerebral death, must be answered at some time in the future. Perhaps wise decisions regarding cerebral death will enable us to resolve these related problems.

References

1. *Adams, A.* Studies on the flat electro-encephalogram in man. Electroenceph. Clin. Neurophysiol. 11:35–41, 1959.
2. *Adams, H.* Letter to editor, "The respirator brain," Arch. Neurol. 33:589–590, 1976.
3. *Adams, R.D., Jequier, M.* The brain death syndrome: hypoxemic panencephalopathy. Schweiz. Med. Wschr. 99:65–73, 1969.
4. *Agnoli, A., Clar, H.E., Magnus, L.* Fehlende Darstellung von Hirngefaessen im Carotisangiogramm infolge intrakranieller Drucksteigerung. Arch. Psychiat. Nervenkr. 213:408–421, 1970.
5. *Ahonen, A., Tolonen, U., Kallanranta, T., Hokkanen, E.* Isotope examination in diagnosis of brain death. Duodecim 95:310–315, 1979.
6. *Alderete, J.F., Jeri, F.R., Richardson, E.P., Sament, S., Schwab, R.S., Young, R.R.* Irreversible coma: A clinical electroencephalographic and neuropathological study. Trans. Amer. Neurol. Ass. 93:16–20, 1968.
7. *Allais, B., Vlahovitch, du Cailar, Delègue, L.* Les critères angiographiques de la mort du cerveau. Anesth. Analg. 28:843–57, 1971.
8. Allegheny County Ad Hoc Committee on Tissue Transplantation. Protocol for the determination of death. Penn. Med. 72:17–20, 1969.
9. *Allen, N., Burkholder, J., Comiscioni, J.* Clinical criteria of brain death. Ann. NY Acad. Sci. 315:70–96, 1978.
10. American Bar Association, Insurance, negligence and compensation law section. Euthanasia—symposium issue. 27 Baylor Law Rev. 1:1–198, 1975.
11. American Electroencephalographic Society. Guidelines in EEG. 30 pp., 1976.
12. *Angstwurm, H., Kugler, J.* Ärztliche Aspekte des Hirntodes und Feststellung des Todeszeitpunktes. Fortschr. Neurol. Psychiatr. 46:291–311, 1978.
13. Anonymous—Device double-checks EEG recordings to determine 'actual moment of death.' NIH Record 23(13):1971 (June 22).
14. Anonymous—EEG signs of death. Brit. Med. J. 2:318, 1968.
15. Anonymous—Le prelevement d'un organe sur un *'mort en survie artificielle.'* Presse. Med. 74:952, 1966.
16. Anonymous—Renal transplantation from mortally injured man. Lancet 2:294, 1963.
17. Anonymous—The moment of death: re Potter (The Times, July 26, 1963). Medicoleg. J. 31:195–196, 1963.
18. Anonymous—Towards a definition of death. J. Med. Soc. New Jersey 64:100–101, 1967.
19. *Aranda, Coddou L.* Muerte cerebral y electroencefalograma. Trabajo experimental. Neurocirurgia 27:174–179, 1969.
20. *Arfel, G.* Stimulations visuelles et silence cérébral. Electroenceph. Clin. Neurophysiol. 23:172–175, 1967.
21. *Arfel, G. Problèmes électroencéphalographiques de la mort.* Masson, Paris: pp. 140, 1970.
22. *Arfel, G.* Problèmes de la mort cérébrale. Med. Leg. Domm. Corpor. (Paris) 3:47–54, 1970.
23. *Arfel, G., Akerman, M., Hertzog, E., Bamberger-Bozo, C.* Données radiologiques, électro-encéphalographiques et isotopiques dans des comas dépassés. Acta Radiol. 13:295–300, 1972.
24. *Arnold, H., Ansorg, P., Voigtsberger, P., Eger, H., Ritter, H.* Beitrag der Pulsationsechoenzephalographie zur Todeszeitbestimmung. Acta Neurochirurgica 27:263–275, 1972.
25. *Arnold, J.D., Zimmerman, T.F., Martin, D.C.* Public attitudes and the diagnosis of death. JAMA 206:1949–1954, 1968.
26. *Asgian, B., Sipos, C., Popoviciu, L.* Dinamica modificarilor poligrafice in comele vascular cerebrale pina la moartea clin-

ica si dupa moartea clinica. Neurologia 18:219–230, 1973.

27. *Ashval, S., Smith, A.J.K., Torres, F., Loken M., Chou, S.N.* Radionuclide bolus angiography; A technique for verification of brain death in infants and children. J. Pediat. 91:722–727, 1977.

28. *Baldy-Moulinier, M., Frèrebeau, P.* Blood flow of the cerebral cortex in intracranial hypertension. Scand. J. Clin. Lab. Invest. Vol. 22: Suppl. 102: VG, 1968.

29. *Baldy-Moulinier, M., Frèrebeau, P.* Cerebral blood flow in cases of coma following severe head injury. In: *Cerebral Flood Flow: Clinical and Experimental Results.* Brock, M., Fieschi, C., Ingvar, D., Lassen, N.A., Schuermann, K. (editors), Springer-Verlag, New York: 216–218, 1969.

30. *Balslev-Jorgensen, P., Heilbrun, M.P., Boysen, G., Rosenklint, A., Jorgensen, E.O.* Cerebral perfusion pressure correlated with regional cerebral blood flow, EEG, and aortocervical arteriography in patients with severe brain disorders progressing to brain death. Europ. Neurol. 8:207–212, 1972.

31. *Bass, M.* Definition of brain death (letter). JAMA 242:1850, 1979.

32. *Baudisch, E., Schleicher, C., Marzoll, I.* The sign of "standing contrast medium column": In craniocerebral trauma (SHT) and for the determination of cerebral death. Radiol. Diagn. (Berl.) 20:253–259, 1979.

33. *Becker, D.P., Robert, C.M., Nelson, J.R., Stern, W.E.* An evaluation of the definition of cerebral death. Neurology 20:459–462, 1970.

34. *Beecher, H.K.* A definition of irreversible coma. Report of the Ad Hoc Committee of the Harvard Medical School to examine the definition of brain death. JAMA 205:337–340, 1968.

35. *Beecher, H.K.* Ethical problems created by the hopelessly unconscious patient. New Eng. J. Med. 278:1425–1530, 1968.

36. *Beecher, H.K.* Definitions of 'life' and 'death' for medical science and practice. Ann. N.Y. Acad. Sci. 169:471–474, 1970.

37. *Bell, J.A., Hodgson, H.J.F.* Coma after cardiac arrest. Brain 97:361–372, 1974.

38. *Bennett, D.R.* The EEG in determination of brain death. Ann. NY Acad. Sci. 315:110–120, 1978.

39. *Bennett, D.R., Hughes, J.R., Korein, J., Merlis, J.K., Suter. C. Atlas of elec-troencephalography in coma and cerebral death.* New York, Raven Press, 244 pp., 1976.

40. *Bennett, D.R., Nord, N.M., Roberts, T.S., Mavor, H.* Prolonged "survival" with flat EEG following cardiac arrest. Electroenceph. Clin. Neurophysiol. 30:94, 1971.

41. *Bental, E., Leibowitz, U.* Flat electroencephalograms during 28 days in a case of 'encephalitis.' Electroenceph. Clin. Neurophysiol. 13:457–460, 1961.

42. *Berger, J.P., Fawer, R.* Cerebrospinal fluid (CSF) lactate and pyruvate in acute neurological situations. In: Lactate in acute conditions. Basel, Karger 115–133, 1979.

43. *Bergen, R.P.* Legal regulation of heart transplants. Dis. Chest 54:352–355, 1968.

44. *Bergquist, E., Bergstrom, J.* Angiography in cerebral death. Acta Radiol. Diag. 12:283–287, 1972.

45. *Berkutov, A.N., Tsybulyak, G.N., Pashkovsky, E.V., Egurnov, N.I., Ivanov, V.V.* Prognosis of severe trauma and diagnosis of brain death in the donor after extraction of the heart for grafting. Eksper Khir. Anestesiol. 2:29–34, 1969.

46. *Bertrand, I., Lhermitte, F., Antoine, B., Ducrot, H.* Nécroses massives de système nerveux central dans une survie artificielle. Rev. Neurol. 101:101–115, 1959.

47. *Bes, A., Arbus, L., Lazorthes, Y., Escande M., Depla, M., Marc Vergne, J.P.* Hemodynamic and metabolic studies in 'coma dépassé': A search for a biological test of death of the brain. In: *Cerebral Blood Flow: Clinical and Experimental Results.* M. Brock, C. Feischi, D.H. Ingvar, N.A. Lassen, K. Schürmann (Eds.), Springer-Verlag, New York, pp. 213–215, 1969.

48. *Bes, A., Geraud, G., Escande, M., Geraud, J.* Difference arterio-veineuse en oxygene dans les comas dépassés. Recherche d'un biologique de la mort du cerveau. Ann Anesth. Franc. 15:80–86, 1974.

49. *Bessert, I., Bushart, W., Horatz, K., Rittmeyer, P.* On the numerical relation between reanimation patients, patients with dissociated brain death and potential organ donors in a reanimation centre. Electroenceph. Clin. Neurophysiol. 29:210–211, 1970.

50. *Bickford, R.G., Dawson, B., Takeshita, H.* Evidence of neurologic death. Electroenceph. Clin. Neurophysiol. 18:513–514, 1965.

51. *Bickford R.G., Sims, J.K., Billinger, T.W., Aung, M.H.* Problems in EEG estimation of brain death and use of com-

puter techniques for their solution. Trauma 12(6):61–95, 1971.

52. *Binnie, C.D., Prior, P.F., Lloyd, D.S.L., Scott, D.F., Margerison, J.H.* Electroencephalographic prediction of fatal anoxic brain damage after resuscitation from cardiac arrest. Brit. Med. J. 4:265–268, 1970.

53. *Biorck, G.* On the definitions of death. World Med. J. 14:137–139, 1967.

54. *Biorck, G.* Thoughts on life and death. Perspect. Biol. Med. 11:527–543, 1968.

55. *Bird, T.D., Plum, F.* Recovery from barbiturate overdose coma with a prolonged isoelectric electroencephalogram. Neurology 18:456–460, 1968.

56. *Black, P.M.* Brain death (first of two parts). N. Engl. J. Med. 299:338–344, 1978.

57. *Black, P.M.* Brain death (second of two parts). N. Engl. J. Med. 299:393–401, 1978.

58. *Black, P. McL.* Criteria of brain death. Postgrad. Med. 57:69–74, 1975.

59. *Bok, S.* Personal directions for care at the end of life. New Eng. J. Med. 295:367–368, 1976.

60. *Boisem, E., Siemkowicz, E.* Six cases of cerebromedullospinal disconnection after cardiac arrest. Lancet 1:1381–1383, 1976.

61. *Boshes, B.* A definition of cerebral death. Ann. Rev. Med. 26:465–470, 1975.

62. *Bots, G.T.A.M., Kramer, W.* Traumatic thrombosis of intracranial arteries and extensive necrosis of the brain developed during reanimation. Acta. Neuropath. 3:416–427, 1964.

63. *Bradac, G.B., Simon, R.S.* Angiography in brain death. J. Neurorad. 7:25–28, 1974.

64. *Braunstein, P., Korein, J., Kricheff, I., Corey, K., Chase, N.* A simple bedside evaluation for cerebral blood flow in the study of cerebral death: A prospective study on 34 deeply comatose patients. Am. J. Roent. Rad. Ther. Nucl. Med. 118:757–767, 1973.

65. *Braunstein, P., Korein, J., Kricheff, I.I., Lieberman, A.* Evaluation of the critical deficit of cerebral circulation using radioactive tracers (Bolus technique). Ann. NY Acad. Sci. 315:143–167, 1978.

66. *Bricolo, A., Benati, A., Mazza C., Bricolo, A.P.* Prolonged isoelectric EEG in a case of post-traumatic coma. Electroenceph. Clin. Neurophysiol. 31:174, 1971.

67. *Brierley, J.B., Adams, J.H., Graham, D.I., Simpson, J.A.* Neocortical death after cardiac arrest. A clinical, neurophysiological, and neuropathological report of two cases. Lancet 2:560–565, 1971.

68. *Brinck, H.P., Gran, L., Larsen, J.L.* Underskelse av fluorescens i retinalkarene for pareising av opphevet cerebral sirkulasjon. Tiddsskr. Nor. Laegeforen 99:364–366, 1979.

69. *Brock, M., Fieschi, C., Ingvar, D., Lassen, N.A., Schürmann, K.* (Eds.) *Cerebral Blood Flow,* Springer-Verlag, pp. 291, 1969.

70. *Brock, M., Schürmann, K., Hadjidimos, A.* Cerebral blood flow and cerebral death. Preliminary report. Acta Neurochir. 20:195–209, 1969.

71. *Brodersen, P., Jorgensen, E.O.* Cerebral blood flow and oxygen uptake, and cerebrospinal fluid biochemistry in severe coma. J. Neurol. Neurosurg. Psychiat. 37:384–391, 1974.

72. *Bronisch, F.W.* Zum Reflexverhalten in Hirntod. Nervenarzt 40:592, 1969.

73. *Brouardel, P.* Death and Sudden Death. Translated by F.L. Benham. Wm. Wood & Co., N.Y., p. 29, 1897.

74. *Bruce, D.A., Langfitt, T.W., Miller, J.D., Schutz, H., Vapalahti, M.P., Stanek, A., Goldberg, H.I.* Regional cerebral blood flow, intracranial pressure, and brain metabolism in comatose patients. J. Neurosurg. 38:131–144, 1973.

75. *Büdingen, H.J., Von Reutern, G.M.* Atraumatische Vorfelddiagnostik des Hirntodes mit der Doppler-Sonographie. Dtsch. Med. Wochenschr. 104:1347–51, 1979.

76. *Buecheler, E., Kaeufer, C.* Karotis und Vertebralisangiographie beim Hirntod. Acta Radiol. Ser. Diagn. 13:301–311, 1972.

77. *Buecheler, E., Kaeufer, C., Duex, A.* Zerebrale Angiographie zur Bestimmung des Hirntodes. Fortschr. Roentgenstr. 113:278–296, 1970.

78. *Burke, G., Halko, A.* Cerebral blood flow studies with sodium pertechnetate Tc 99m and the scintillation camera. JAMA 204:109–114, 1968.

79. *Burns, J.M., Hamlon, J.S.* Minnesota "brain death" legislation: a step forward . . . or backward? Minn. Med. 62:273–277, 1979.

80. *Bushart, W., Rittmeyer, P.* Elektroencephalographische Verlaufsueberwachung und Kriterien der irreversiblen Hirnschae-

digung in der Intensivpflege. Verh. Deutsch. Ges. Inn. Med. 74:865–868, 1968.
81. *Bushart, W., Rittmeyer, P.* Kriterien der irreversiblen Hirnschaedigung bei Intensivbehandlung: Elektroenzephalographische und klinische Verlaufsueberwachung. Med. Klin. 64:184–193, 1969.
82. *Busse, O., Vogelsang, H.* Transfemorale zerebrale Panarteriographie zur Bestimmung des Hirntodes. Fortschr. Röntgenstr. 121:639–634, 1974.
83. *Butcher, P.H.* Management of the relatives of patients with brain death. Int. Anesthesiol. Clin. 17:327–332, 1979.
84. *Byrne, P.A., O'Reilly, S., Quay, P.M.* Brain death—an opposing viewpoint. JAMA 242:1985–1990, 1979.
85. *Cahn, J., Mathis, P., Herold, M., Alano, J., Van Holten, I., Barre, N.* Effects of acute anoxia on EEG and brain metabolism in the rabbit and dog. In *Cerebral anoxia and the Electroencephalogram.* Meyer, J.S., Gastaut, H., editors. C.C Thomas, Springfield, Ill. 89–104, 1961.
86. Canadian Medical Association Statement on death. Canad. Med. Ass. J. 99:1266–1267, 1968.
87. *Capron, A.M., Kass, L.R.* A statutory definition of the standards for determining human death; an appraisal and a proposal. Univ. Penna. Law Review, 121:87–118, 1972.
88. *Carr, W.* Theological reflections on death. N. Carolina Med. J. 28:461–464, 1967.
89. *Carroll, T.J.* Cerebral death: theological considerations. Unpublished manuscript, presented at meeting of the American Association of Neurological Surgeons, Cleveland, Ohio, April 15, 1969.
90. *Carter, F., Chevet, D., LePolles, R., Launois, B.* La fonction renale des comas dépassés. Ann. Anesth. Franc. 15:21–26, 1974.
91. *Castelan, D.S.* Cerebral death (letter). Heart Lung 7:1066, 1978.
92. *Celsus, A.C* In re medicina. Editio princeps, Florence, 1478.
93. *Chatrian, G.E., White, L.E., Shaw, C.M.* EEG pattern resembling wakefulness in unresponsive decerebrate state following traumatic brainstem infarct. Electroenceph. Clin. Neurophysiol. 16:285–289, 1964.
94. *Chatterjee, S.N., Payne, J.E., Berne, T.V.* Difficulties in obtaining kidneys from potential postmortem donors. JAMA 232:822–824, 1975.

95. *Chiang, J., Kowada, M., Ames, A., Wright, R.L., Majno, G.* Cerebral ischemia. III. Vascular changes. Amer J. Path. 52:455–476, 1968.
96. *Chukhrova, V.A., Popova, L.M.* Electroencephalographic signs of brain death after respiratory resuscitation. Zh. Nevropatol. Psikhiatr. 78:659–663, 1978.
97. *Clar, H.E., Agnoli, A., Magnus, L.* Angiographische Befund bei intracraniellem Kreislaufstillstand infolge erhöhten Hirndruches. Acta Radiol. 13:312–317, 1972.
98. *Cochs, J., Buetas, E., Cobos, P.* Conveniencia de modificacion del concepto legal de muerte. Rev. Esp. Anestesiol. Reanin. 25:98–113, 1978.
99. Collaborative Study. "An appraisal of the criteria of cerebral death—a summary statement." JAMA 237:982–986, 1977.
100. *Connor, R.C.R.* Heart damage associated with intracranial lesions. Brit. Med. J. 3:29–31, 1968.
101. Council for International Organizations of Medical Sciences (CIOMS): Concerning heart transplantation. Presse. Med. 76:1390, 1968.
102. Conseil National de l'Ordre des Medecins: The removal of an organ from a patient being kept alive artificially. Presse. Med. 74:952, 1966.
103. *Crafoord, C.C.* Cerebral death and the transplantation era. Dis. Chest 55:141–145, 1969.
104. *Cranford, R.E.* Brain death. Concept and criteria. Minn. Med. 61:600–603, 1978.
105. *Cranford, R.E.* Minnesota Medical Association Criteria. Brain death. Concept and criteria. Minn. Med. 61:561–563, 1978.
106. *Cravioto, H., Silberman, J., Feigin, I.* A clinical and pathologic study of akinetic mutism. Neurology 10:10–21, 1960.
107. *Creighton, H.* What is death and who determines it? Superv. Nurse 10:17–18, 74–75, 1979.
108. *Crow, H.J., Winter, A.* Serial electrophysiological studies (EEG, EMG, ERG, evoked responses) in a case of 3 months survival with flat EEG following cardiac arrest. Electroenceph. Clin. Neurophysiol. 27:332-333, 1969.
109. *Curran, W.J.* Public Health and the law: the legal meaning of death. Amer. J. Public Health 58:1965–1966, 1968.
110. *Curran, W.J.* Legal and medical death—Kansas takes the first step. New Eng. J. Med. 284:260–261, 1971.
111. *Curran, W.J.* Settling the medicological

issues concerning brain death statutes: matters of legal ethics and judicial precedent. N. Engl. J. Med. 299:31-32, 1978.

112. *Curran, W.J.* The brain-death concept; judicial acceptance in Massachusetts. N. Engl. J. Med. 298:1008–1009, 1978.

113. *Cushing, H.* Some experimental and clinical observations concerning states of increased intracranial tension. Am. J. Med. Sci. 124:375–400, 1902.

114. *David, E., Marx, I., David, H.* Das Ultrastrukturelle Bild der Nervenzelle in verschiedenen Regionen des Meerschweinchengehirns im Verlauf der postmortalen Autolyse. Exp. Path. 5:98–106, 1971.

115. *Decker, K., Kunkel, B.* Zerebrale Angiographie und Hirntod. Fortschr. Röntgenstr. 118:617–623, 1973.

116. *Deraux, J.P. In Gros, C.* Les critères circulatoires et biologiques de la mort du cerveau. Neuro-Chirurgie, 18:9–48 (p. 26), 1972.

117. *DeRougemont, J., Barge, M., Benabid, A.L.* L'égalisation des pressions intracranienne et arterielle systémique dans les états de mort encéphalique. Ann Anesth. Franc. 15:117–121, 1974.

118. *DeRougemont, J., Barge, M., Benabid, A.L., Cordeiro, A.* Les arrèts circulatoires encéphaliques: Données apportées par l'enregistrement comparatif des pressions arterielle et intracranienne. Neuro-Chirurgie 15:584–586, 1969.

119. *Despland, P.A., DeCrousaz, G.* L'apport de l'ultrasonographic Doppler au diagnostic de la mort cérébrale. Schw. Med. Wsch. 104:1454–1459, 1974.

120. *deVlieger, M., Crezee, P., van Dongen, K.J.* Enkele technische aspecten van de diagnostiek van hernesdood. Ned. Tijdschr. Geneeskd. 122:33–38, 1978.

121. *Doering, H.J., Olbrisch, R.R., Schrader, J., Lang, H.* Elektrocorticogramm, Bestandspotential des Gehirns und energiereiche Phosphatfraktionen der Hirnrinde bei Narkoticum-Ueberdosierung, Ischaemie und Cyanidvergiftung. Pflueger Arch. 319:12–35, 1970.

122. *Dolce, G., Sannita, W.* A CNV-like negative shift in deep coma. Electroenceph. Clin. Neurophysiol. 34:647–650, 1973.

123. *Drory, Y., Ouaknine, G., Kosary, I.Z., Kellerman, J.J.* Electrocardiographic findings in brain death; description and presumed mecahnism. Chest 67:425–432, 1975.

124. *Duven, H.E., Kollrack, H.W.* Areflexie: Kein obligates Symptom bei diz-

zoziiertem Hirntod. Deutsch Med. Wschr. 95:1346–1348, 1970.

125. *Ectors, L.* Paralysie vasculaire cerebrale. Acta. Neurol. Belg. 69:33–50, 1969.

126. Editorial, Uniform Brain Death Act. Neurology (Minneap.), 29:417–418, 1979.

127. *Edwards, H.A., Benstead, J.G., Brown, K., Makary, A.Z., Menon, N.K.* Apparent death with accidental hypothermia. A case report. Brit. J. Anaesth. 42:906–908, 1970.

128. *Eklöf, B., Siesjö, B.K.* Cerebral blood flow and cerebral energy state. Acta Physiol. Scand. 82:409–411, 1971.

129. *Epstein, F.H.* No, it's our duty to keep patients alive. Med. Economics 4:97–101, 1973.

130. *Feldman, M.H.* Physiological observations in chronic case of "locked-in" syndrome. Neurology 21:459–478, 1971.

131. *Feild, J.R., Leo, L., McBurney, R.F.* Complications of 1000 brachial arteriograms. J. Neurosurg. 36:324–332, 1972.

132. *Feild, J.R., Robertson, J.T., De-Saussure, R.L.* Complications of cerebral angiography in 2000 consecutive cases. J. Neurosurg. 19:775-781, 1962.

133. *Ferrillo, F., Giunta, F., Rivano, C., Rodriguez, G., Rosadini, G., Rossi, G.F., Sannita, W., Siania, C., Tuella, G., Zattoni, J.* Analysis of the spontaneous and evoked cerebral electrical activity in deep coma and in "cerebral death." Electroenceph. Clin. Neurophysiol 31:174, 1971.

134. *Findji, F., Gaches, J., Houtteville, J.P., Creissard, P., Caliskan, A.* Enregistrements éléctroencéphalographiques corticaux, transcorticaux, et souscorticaux dans dix cas de coma profond ou dépassé (note préliminaire). Neurochirurgia 13:211–219, 1970.

135. *Fischgold, H., Mathis, P.* Obnubilations, comas et stupeurs. Masson & Cie, Paris, 125 pp., 1959.

136. *Flatmark, A., Bondevik, H.* The brain death kidney donor. Scan. J. Urol. Nephrol. 8:235–239, 1974.

137. *Frèrebeau, P.* La circulation cérébrale du coma dépassé. Ann. Anesth. Franc. 15 (special III): 34–40, 1974.

138. *Frumin, M.S., Epstein, R.M., Cohen, G.* Apneic oxygenation in man. Anesthesiol. 20:789–798, 1959.

139. *Fuchs, E.C., Schneider, H.* Demonstration of early capillary lesions in the brain by means of artificial reperfusion. Adv. Neurol. 20:503–510, 1978.

140. *Fujimoto, T.* "Brain Death" and vital phenomena; autopsy findings in cases

maintained on a respirator for a prolonged period. Jap. J. Clin. Med. 31:700–706, 1973.

141. *Gaches, J., Caliskan, A., Findji, F., LeBeau, J.* Contribution à l'étude du coma dépassé et de la mort cérébrale. Sem. Hôp. Paris 46:1487–1497, 1970.

142. *Garcia, J.J., Kámijyo, Y.* Cerebral infarction. Evolution of histopathological changes after occlusion of a middle cerebral artery in primates. J. Neuropath. Exp. Neurol. 33:408–420, 1974.

143. *Géraud, J., Bès, A., Rascol, A., Delpla, M., Marc-Vergnes, J.P., Escande, M., Géraud, G.* Etude hémodynamique et métabolique de certains comas, notamment comas apoplectiques et comas dépassés. Rev. Neurol. 121:74–88, 1969.

144. *Gerin, C., Merli, S.* La mort et les transplantations d'organes. La constatation de la mort. Zacchia 7:1–52, 1971.

145. *Gerlach, J.* Die Definition des Todes in ihrer heutigen Problematik fuer Medizin und Rechtlehre. Arztrecht 6:83–86, 1968.

146. *Gerlach, G.* Individualtod, Partialtod, Vita reducta. Münch. Med. Wschr. 110:980–983, 1968.

147. *Gerlach, G.* Gehirntod und totaler Tod. Münch. Med. Wschr. 111:732–736, 1969.

148. German Surgical Society. Definition of the signs and time of death. Statement by the Commission on Reanimation and Organ Transplantation. German Med. Monthly 13:359, 1968.

149. *Gerstenbrand, F.* Das traumatische apallische Syndrom. Springer-Verlag, New York. 344 pp., 1967.

150. *Gerstenbrand, F., Luecking, C.H.* Die akuten traumatischen Hirnstammschaeden. Arch. Psychiat. Nervenkr. 213:264–281, 1970.

151. *Gilder, S.S.B.* Twenty-second World Medical Assembly: death and the W.M.A. Brit. Med. J. 3:493–494, 1968.

152. *Gilman, L.S., Gilman, A.* The pharmacological basis of therapeusis. London. The MacMillan and Co., 4th Edit. 1970, XX + 1794 pp., Chap. 25, p. 524.

153. *Girard, P.F., Tommasi, M., Trillet, M.* Les lesions anatomiques de l'encéphalopathie posttraumatique (comas prolongés et 'morts du cerveau'). Acta Neuropath. 2:313–327, 1963.

154. *Goertchen, R., Willbrandt, D., Mesewinkel, J.* Zur Neuropathologie des atraumatischen apallischen Symptomkomplexes und des intravitalen Hirntodes bei Inten-

sivtherapie. Z. Aerztl. Forbild (Jena) 72:499–505, 1978.

155. *Goldensohn, E.S.* The relationship of the EEG to the clinical examination in determining brain death. Ann. NY Acad. Sci. 315:137–142, 1978.

156. *Goodman, J.M., Mishkin, F.S., Dyken, M.* Determination of brain death by isotope angiography. JAMA 209:1869–1872, 1969.

157. *Gould,* Blackiston's Gould's Medical Dictionary. Blackiston 1828 pp., 1972.

158. *Grass, E.R.* Technological aspects of electroencephalography in the determination of death. Amer. J. EEG Technol. 9:77–90, 1969.

159. *Green, J.B., Lauber, A.* Return of EEG activity after electrocerebral silence: Two case reports. J. Neurol. Neurosurg. Psychiatry 35:103–107, 1972.

160. *Greenfield, J.G., Meyer, A.* General pathology of the nerve cell and neuroglia, In: Greenfield's Neuropathology 2nd Ed. Baltimore, Williams and Wilkins pp. 29–34, 1963.

161. *Greitz, T., Gordon, E., Kolmodin, G., Widen, L.* Aortocranial and carotid angiography in determination of brain death. Neuroradiology 5:13–19, 1973.

162. *Grenvik, A., Powner, D.J., Snyder, J.V., Jastremski, M.S., Babcock, R.A., Loughhead, M.G.* Cessation of therapy in terminal illness and brain death. Crit. Care Med. 6:284–291, 1978.

163. *Gros, C.* Less critères circulatoires et biologiques de la mort du cerveau. (à l'éxclusion des problèmes cliniques et électroencéphalographiques). Neurochirurgie 18:9–48, 1972.

164. *Gros, C., Vlahovitch, B., Frèrebeau, P., Kuhner, A., Billet, M., Sahut, G., Gavand, G.* Critères artériographiques des comas dépassés en neurochirurgie. Neurochirurgie 15:477–486, 1969.

165. *Grunnet, L., Paulson, G.* Pathological changes in irreversible brain death. Diseases of the Nervous System 32:690–694, 1971.

166. *Habel, G., Schneider, I.* Feststellung des Hirntodes unter besonderer Berüchsichtigung des jungen Kindesalters. Zbl. Chir. 100:421–426, 1975.

167. *Hadjidimos, A.A., Brock, M., Baum, P., Schurmann, K.* Cessation of cerebral blood flow in total irreversible loss of brain function. In: M. Brock, C. Fieschi, D.H. Ingvar, N.A. Lassen, K. Schurmann (Eds.)

Cerebral Blood Flow: Clinical and Experimental Results, Springer-Verlag, New York, pp. 209–212, 1969.

168. *Hager, H.* Die frühen Alterationen des Nervengewebes nach Hypoxidose und die fortgeschrittene Nekrose im elektronenmikroskopischen Bild. in Proc. 5th Intern. Congr. Neuropath. Leuthy, F. and Bischoff, A. (Eds.) Excerpta Medica Foundation, Amsterdam:64–78, 1966.

169. *Haider, I., Oswald, I.* Electroencephalographic investigation in acute drug poisoning. Electroenceph. Clin. Neurophysiol. 29:105, 1970.

170. *Haider, I., Oswald, I., Matthew, H.* EEG signs of death. Brit. Med. J. 3:314, 1968.

171. *Halley, M.M., Harvey, W.F.* Definition of death. New Eng. J. Med. 279:834, 1968.

172. *Halley, M.M., Harvey, W.F.* Law-medicine comment: definitions of death. J. Kansas Med. Soc. 69:280–282, 1968.

173. *Halley, M.M., Harvey, W.F.* Medical vs legal definitions of death. JAMA 204:423–425, 1968.

174. *Hamlin, H.* Life or death by EEG. JAMA 190:112–114, 1964.

175. *Hamlon, J.S., Burns, J.M.* Minnesota "brain death" legislation: a step forward . . . or backward? II. Defining "brain death." Minn. Med. 62:363–365, 372, 1979.

176. *Hamner, R.T.* Legal death—can it be defined? J. Med. Ass. Alabama. 38:610–614, 1969.

177. *Harp, J.R.* Criteria for the determination of death. Anesthesiology 40:391–397, 1974.

178. *Hass, W.K., Ransohoff, J., Wood, D.H., Wald, A.* Continuous *in vivo* monitoring by mass spectrometry of human blood gases and cerebral blood flow. Trans. Amer. Neurol. Ass. 95:255–257, 1970.

179. *Hauerwas, S.* Religious concepts of brain death and associated problems. Ann. NY Acad. Sci. 315:329–338, 1978.

180. *Heiskanen, O.* Cerebral circulatory arrest caused by acute increase of intracranial pressure. Acta Scand. Neurol. 40: Suppl. 17:1–57, 1964.

181. *Heiss, W.D.* Cerebral blood flow and brain stem lesion. Z. Neurol. 203:197–209, 1972.

182. *Held, K., Gottstein, U.* Durchblutung und Stoffwechsel des menschlichen Gehirns nach akuter cerebraler Ischamie. Verh. Dtsch. Ges. Inn. Med. 78:665–668, 1972.

183. *Herrick, M.K., Agamanolis, D.F.* Displacement of cerebellar tissue into spinal canal. A component of the respirator brain syndrome. Arch. Path. 99:565–571, 1975.

184. *Hicks, R.G., Torda, T.A.* The vestibulo-ocular (caloric) reflex in the diagnosis of cerebral death. Anaesth. Intensive Care 7:169–173, 1979.

185. *Hirsh, H.L.* Brain death—medical trial. Tech. Quart. 377–405,1975.

186. *Hoedt-Rasmussen, K.* Regional cerebral blood flow. The intra-arterial injection method. Acta. Neurol. Scand. 43: Suppl. 27, 1967.

187. *Hoffman, A.C., Van Cura, M.X.* Death—the five brain criteria. Med. Trial Tech. Q. 24:377–407, 1978.

188. *Hogue, J.M.* Brain cells from human fetuses and infant, cultured in vitro after death of the individuals. Anat. Rec. 108:457–476, 1950.

189. *Holmdahl, M.H.* Pulmonary uptake of oxygen, acid-base metabolism, and circulation during prolonged apnea. Acta Chirurg. Scand. Suppl. 212, 128 pp., 1956.

190. *Homan, R.W.* Ethical, legal, and medical aspects of brain death: a review and proposal. Tex. Med. 75:36–43, 1979.

191. *Horan, D.J.* Euthanasia and brain death: ethical and legal consideration. Ann. NY Acad. Sci. 315:363–375, 1978.

192. *Horwitz, N., Dunsmore, R.* Some factors influencing the nonvisualization of the internal carotid artery by angiography. J. Neurosurg. 13:155–164, 1956.

193. *Hossmann, K.A.* Cortical steady potential, impedance, and excitability changes during and after total ischemia of cat brain. Exp. Neurol. 32:163–175, 1971.

194. *Hossmann, K.A., Kleihues, P.* Reversibility of ischemic brain damage. Arch. Neurol. 29:375–384, 1973.

195. *Hossmann, K.A., Sahaki, S., Kimoto, K.* Cerebral uptake of glucose and oxygen in the cat brain after prolonged ischemia. Stroke 7:301–304, 1976.

196. *Hossmann, K.A., Sato, K.* Effect of ischemia on the function of the sensorimotor cortex in cat. Electroenceph. Clin. Neurophysiol. 30:535–545, 1971.

197. *Houts, M.* New horizons for the EEG; the diagnosis of death. Trauma 12(6):1–12, 1971.

198. *Hoyer, S., Wawersik, J.* Untersuchungen der Hirndurchblutung und des Hirnstoffwechsels beim Decerebrationssyn-

drom. Legenbecks Arch. Chir. 322:602–605, 1968.

199. *Hughes, J.R.* Limitations of the EEG in coma and brain death. Ann. NY Acad. Sci. 315:121–136, 1978.

200. *Hurwitz, B.S., Wolfson, S.K.* Brain lactate in anoxia and hypothermia: relationship to brain viability. Exp. Neurol. 23:426–434, 1969.

201. *Ibe, K.* Clinical and pathophysiological aspects of the intravital brain death. Electroenceph. Clin. Neurophysiol. 30:272, 1971.

202. *Icard. S.* Du danger de la morte apparente. Presse Med. 2:521–525, 1904.

203. *Ingvar, D.H.* EEG and cerebral circulation in the apallic syndrome and akinetic mutism. Electroenceph. Clin. Neurophysiol. 30:272–273, 1971.

204. *Ingvar, D. H., Brun, A., Johansson, L., Samuelsson, S. M.* Survival after severe cerebral anoxia with destruction of the cerebral cortex: the apallic syndrome. Ann. N.Y. Acad. Sci. 315, 184–214, 1979

205. *Ingvar, D.H., Lassen, N.A., Siesjo, B.K., Skinhoj, E.* Cerebral Blood Flow and Cerebro-Spinal Fluid. Scand. J. Clin. Lab. Invest. 22: Suppl. 102, 1968.

206. *Ingvar. D.H., Sourander, P.* Destruction of the reticular core of the brain stem. A patho-anatomical followup of a case of coma of three years' duration. Arch. Neurol. 23:1–8, 1970.

207. *Ingvar, D.H., Widen, L.* Death of the brain—man's death. Lakartidningen 64:4899–4903, 1967.

208. *Ingvar, D.H., Widen, L.* Brain death—Summary of a symposium. Lakartidningen 34:3804–3814, 1972.

209. Institute of Society, Ethics and the Life Sciences. Task Force on Death and Dying, Refinements in criteria for the determination of death: an appraisal. JAMA 221:48–54, 1970.

210. *Ishiguro, T., Hayashi, M., Kamisasa, A.* The brain stem and the spinal functions, at brain death and similar states. Psychiat. Neurol. Jap. 75:481–98, 540–41, 1973.

211. *Ivan, L.P.* Irreversible brain damage and related problems; pronouncement of death. J. Amer. Geriat. Soc. 18:816–822, 1970.

212. *Ivan, L.P.* Spinal reflexes in cerebral death. Neurol. 23:650–652, 1973.

213. *Jacob, H.* Patterns of CNS vulnerability. CNS tissue and cellular pathology in hypoxaemic states. In: *Selective Vulnerability of the Brain in Hypoxaemia: A Symposium.* Schade, J.P. and McMenemey, W.H. (Eds.) Blackwell Scientific Publications, Oxford: 153–163, 1963.

214. *Jährig, K.* Grenzen der Lebenserhaltung beim Neugeborenen. Zur Bestimmung des Hirntodes in den Neonatalzeit, Kinderärztl. Prax. 47:65–70, 1979.

215. *Jastremski, M., Powner, D., Snyder, J., Smith, J., Grenvik, A.* Problems in brain death determination. Forensic Sci. 11:201–212, 1978.

216. *Jellinger, K.* Zur Morphologie komatoeser und postkomatoeser Encephalopathien. Excerpta Medica Intern. Congr. No. 100, 3–20, 1966.

217. *Jellinger, K.* Zur Neuropathologie des Komas und postkomatoeser Encephalopathien. Wien klin. Wschr. 80:505–517, 1968.

218. *Jennett, B.* Irrecoverable brain damage after resuscitation: brain death and other syndromes. Resuscitation 5:49–52, 1976.

219. *Jennett, B., Plum, F.* Persistent vegetative state after brain damage—A syndrome in search of a name. Lancet 1:734–737, 1972.

220. *Jonkman, E.J.* Cerebral death and the isoelectric EEG. Electroenceph. Clin. Neurophysiol. 27:215, 1969.

221. *Jorgensen, E.O.* The EEG during severe barbiturate intoxication. Acta. Neurol. Scand. 46:281, 1970.

222. *Jorgensen, E.O.* Spinal man after brain death. Acta Neurochir. 28:259–273, 1973.

223. *Jorgenseñ, E.O.* Requirements for recording the EEG at high sensitivity in suspected brain death. Electroenceph. Clin. Neurophysiol. 36:65–69, 1974.

224. *Jorgensen, E.O.* EEG without detectable cortical activity and cranial nerve areflexia as parameters of brain death. Electroenceph. Clin. Neurophysiol. 36:70–75, 1974.

225. *Jorgensen, P.B.* Clinical deterioration prior to brain death related to progressive intracranial hypertension. Acta. Neurochir. 28:29–40, 1973.

226. *Jorgensen, P.B.* Brain Death. Cerebral appearance of inhaled hydrogen in the diagnosis of cerebral circulatory arrest. Acta Neurochir. 30:187–193, 1974.

227. *Jorgensen, P.B., Jorgensen, E.O., Rosenklint, A.* Brain death pathogenesis and diagnosis. Acta Neurol. Scand. 49:355–367, 1973.

228. *Jouvet, M.* Diagnostic electro-sous-cortico-graphique de la mort du système nerveux central au cours de certains comas.

Electroenceph. Clin. Neurophysiol. 11:805–808, 1959.

229. *Juul-Jensen, P.* Criteria of Brain Death: Selection of Donors for Transplantation. Munksgaard, Copenhagen. 57 pp., 1970.

230. *Kaeufer, C.* Die Bestimmung des Todeszeitpunktes. Fortschr. Med. 90:1125–1126, 1972.

231. *Kaefer, C.* Criteria of cerebral death. Minn. Med. 56:321–324, 1973.

232. *Kaeufer, C., Penin, H.* Todeszeitbestimmung beim dissoziierten Hirntod: Klinische und elektroenzephalographische Kriterien. Deutsch Med. Wschr. 93:679–684, 1968.

233. *Kaeufer, C., Penin, H., Deux, A., Kersting, G., Schneider, H., Kubicki, S.* Zerebraler Zirkulationsstillstand bei Hirntod durch Hypoxydosen. Fortschr. Med. 87:713–717, 1969.

234. *Kass, L.R.* Death as an event: a commentary on Robert Morison. Science 173:698–702, 1971.

235. *Kaste, M., Hillbom, M., Palo, J.* Diagnosis and management of brain death. Br. Med. J. 1:525–527, 1979.

236. *Katsurada, K., Susimoto, T.* Oxygen tension of the blood of the internal jugular vein and cerebrospinal fluid in patients with brain injury. Brain Nerve (Tokyo) 23:163–171, 1971.

237. *Kawai, S.* Clinical and experimental studies on the process of brain death by repetitive evoked electromyography. J. Nara Med. Ass. 24:273–300, 1973.

238. *Keane, J.R.* Blinking to sudden illumination. A brainstem reflex present in neocortical death. Arch. Neurol. 36:52–53, 1979.

239. *Kendall, M.G.* Rank correlation methods. New York, Hafner Publishing Co. 3rd Ed. VII + 199 pp., 1962.

240. *Kero, P., Antila, K., Ylitalo, V., V'alim'aki, I.* Decreased heart rate variation in decerebration syndrome: quantitative clinical criterion of brain death? Pediatrics 62:307–311, 1978.

241. *Kety, S.S.* The cerebral circulation. Handbook of Physiology, Sect. I, Neurophysiology 3(71):1751–1760, 1960.

242. *Ketz, E.* Bewusstseinsstörungen in der Neurologie. Praxis 59(30):1081–1089, 1970.

243. *Ketz, E.* Beitrag zum Problem des Hirntodes (Beobachtungen an 100 Fällen von totalem Hirnfunktionsausfall) Schw. Arch. Neurol. Neurochirurgie u. Psychiat. 110:205–221, 1972.

244. *Kevorkian, J.* Rapid and accurate ophthalmoscopic determination of circulatory arrest. JAMA 164:1660–1664, 1957.

245. *Kimura, J., Gerber, H.W., McCormick, W.F.* The isoelectric electroencephalogram. Significance in establishing death in patients maintained on mechanical respirators. Arch. Intern. Med. 121:511–517, 1968.

246. *Kindt, G.W.* Autoregulation of spinal cord blood flow. In: Cerebral Blood Flow and Intracranial Pressure. Proc. 5th International Symposium, European Neurology 6:19–23, 1971–2.

247. *Kirschbaum, R.J., Carollo, V.J.* Reversible isoelectric EEG in barbiturate coma. JAMA 212:1215, 1970.

248. *Kjeldsberg, C.R.* Respirator brain. In: Minckler. J. (Ed.) Pathology of the Nervous System. McGraw-Hill Book Company, New York. 3:2952–2961, 1972.

249. *Kohlhaas, M.* Zur Feststellung des Todeszeitpunktes Verstorbener. Deutsch Med. Wschr. 93:412–414, 1968.

250. *Korein, J.* On cerebral, brain and systemic death. Current concepts of cerebralvascular disease. Stroke 8:9–14, 1973.

251. *Korein, J., Ed.* Brain death: interrelated medical and social issues, Ann. NY Acad. Sci. 315:1–454, 1978.

252. *Korein, J.* Brain death: interrelated medical and social issues. Preface, Ann. NY Acad. Sci. 315:1–5, 1978.

253. *Korein, J.* Brain death: interrelated medical and social issues. Terminology, definitions, and usage, Ann. NY Acad. Sci. 315:6–18, 1978.

254. *Korein, J.* The problem of brain death: development and history, Ann. NY Acad. Sci. 315:19–38, 1978.

255. *Korein, J., Braunstein, P., Kricheff, I., Lieberman, A., Chase, N.* Radioisotopic bolus technique as a test to detect circulatory deficit associated with cerebral death. Circulation 51:924–939, 1975.

256. *Korein, J., Maccario, M.* On the diagnosis of cerebral death: a prospective study on 55 patients to define irreversible coma. Clinical Electroencephalography 2:178–199, 1971.

257. *Kowada, M., Ames, A., Majno, G., Wright, R.L.* Cerebral ischemia. I. An improved experimental method for study: cardiovascular effects and demonstration of an early vascular lesion in the rabbit. J. Neurosurg. 28:150–157, 1968.

258. *Kramer, W.* From reanimation to deanimation. Acta. Neurol. Scand. 39:139–153, 1963.

259. *Kramer, W.* Progressive posttraumatic encephalopathy during reanimation. Acta. Neurol. Scan. 40:249–258, 1964.
260. *Kramer, W.* Extensive necrosis of the brain development during reanimation. Proc. 5th Intern. Congr. Neuropath., Excerpta Medica Intern. Congr. Series No. 100:33–45, 1966.
261. *Kramer, W.* Die Schwelle zum Tode. Probleme der Wiederbelebung. Arztl Prax. 20:1091, 1107–1111, 1968.
262. *Kramer, W.* Acute lethal intracranial hypertension. Clinical and experimental observations. Psychiat. Neurol. Neurochir. 73:243–255, 1970.
263. *Kramer, W., Tuynman, J.A.* Acute intracranial hypertension—an experimental investigation. Brain Res. 6:686–705, 1967.
264. *Kricheff, I.I., Pinto, R.S., George, A.E., Braunstein, P., Korein, J.* Angiographic findings in brain death, Ann. NY Acad. Sci. 315:168–183, 1978.
265. *Krözl, W., Scherzer, E.* Die Bestimmung des Todeszeitpunktes. Kongress in der Wiener Hofburg, Mai 1972. Allg. Unfallvers. Anstalt, Vienna. 378 pp. 1973.
266. *Kuhne, D., Arnold, H.* Zur neuroradiologischen Diagnose des zerebralen Kreislaufstillstandes. Med. Welt. 29:1678–1679, 1978.
267. *Kurtz, D., Cornette, M., Tempe, J.D., Mantz, J.M.* Prognostic value of the EEG following reversible cardiac arrest. From 90 cases. Electroenceph. Clin. Neurophysiol. 29:530–531, 1970.
268. *Kurtz, D., Cornette, M., Tempe, J.D., Mantz, J.M.* Interet de l'EEG dans les suites d'arret cardiaque reversible. Acta Neurol. Belg. 70:213–227, 1970.
269. *Kurtz, D., Mantz, J.M., Tempe, J.D., Feuerstein, J.* Silence électrique cérébral prolongé et reversible: A propos de trois observations. Rev Neurol. 115:423–428, 1966.
270. *Laborit, G., Legrand, A., Soufir, J.C.* Le liquide cephalorachidien des comas dépassés. Ann. Anesth. Franc. 15:48–60, 1974.
271. *Lamoureux, F., Chartrand, R., Copti, M., Guimond, J., Bissoon-Doyal, D.* Le diagnostic du mort cérébrale par une méthode radioisotopique simple et rapide, Union Med. Can. 107:41–46, 1978.
272. *Langfitt, T.W., Kassell, N.F.* Nonfilling of cerebral vessels during angiography. Correlation with intracranial pressure. Acta. Neurochir. 14:96–104, 1966.

273. *Lanner, G., Argyropoulos, G.* Neuere Aspekte für die Bestimmung des zerebralen Todes. Wien Klin. Wschr. 85:99–102, 1973.
274. *Lausberg, G.* Der Verlust der Temperaturregulation beim zentralen Tod: reversibel? Deutsch Med. Wschr. 95:1301–1303, 1970.
275. *Lausberg, G.* Die Bedeutung zentraler Temperaturregulationsstörhungen zur Therapie und Prognose schwerer gedeckter Schädelhirnverletzungen. Hefte Unfallheilk. 107:209–213, 1970.
276. *Lazorthes, Y. In Gros, C.* Les Critères circulatoires et biologiques et de la mort du cerveau Neuro-Chirurgie. 18:9–48. p.26, 1972.
277. *Lazorthes, Y., Bes, A. In Gros, C.* Les critères circulatoires et biologiques de la mort du cerveau. Neuro-Chirurgie. 18:9–48. p. 26–27, 1972.
278. *Lecuire, J., Deruty, R., Dechaume, J.P., Lapras, C.* Considerations actuelles sur d'évolution lointaine des traumatismes craniocérébraux graves avec coma prolongé. Neuro-Chirurgie 19:271–277, 1973.
279. *Lecuire, J., Rougemont, J. de, Descottes, J., Jouvet, M.* Données concernant les arrêts circulatoires encéphaliques. Intérêt de test à l'atropine, Neuro-Chir. 8, 158–167, 1962.
280. *Leenstra-Borsje, H., Boonstra, S., Blokzijl, E.J., Notermans, S.L.H.* A retrospective investigation of the clinical symptoms and course of patients with a complete or incomplete isoelectric EEG. Electroenceph. Clin. Neurophysiol. 27:215, 1969.
281. *Leksell, L.* Echoencephalography. Act. Chir. Scand. 110:(3) 301, 1955.
282. *Lepetit, J.M., Pefferkorn, J.P* Aspects de l'écho-encéphalogramme au cours de l'évolution des comas spécialement au stade "coma dépassé" In: *"Reanimation et ethique medicale,"* edited by Mollaret and Vermujp, Paris, Arnette 31–38, 1970.
283. *Lepetit, J.M., Pefferkorn, J.P., Dany, A.* Echographie pulsatile et perte irreversible des fonctions cérébrales. Ann. Anesth. Franc. 15:101–108, 1974.
284. *Levin, P., Kinnell, J.* Successful cardiac resuscitation despite prolonged silence of EEG. Arch. Intern. Med. 117:557–560, 1966.
285. *Levine, J.E., Becker, D., Chun, T.* Reversal of incipient brain death from head-injury apnea at the scene of accidents (letter), N. Engl. J. Med. 301:109, 1979.

286. *Levy-Alcover, M.A., Babinet, P.* Chronological relationship between establishment of clinical irreversible coma and persistence of minimal EEG activity in nine cases. Electroenceph. Clin. Neurophysiol. 29:531–532, 1970.

287. *Liebhardt, E.W., Wuermeling, H.B.* Juristisch und medizinisch-naturwissenschaftliche Begriffsbildung und die Feststellung des Todeszeitpunktes. Münch. Med. Wschr. 110:1661–1665, 1968.

288. *Lindenberg, R.* Patterns of CNS vulnerability in acute hypoxaemia, including anaesthesia accidents. In: *Selective Vulnerability of the Brain in Hypoxaemia: A Symposium.* Schade, J.P. and McMenemey, W.H. (Eds.) Blackwell Scientific Publications, Oxford: 189–209, 1963.

289. *Lindenberg, R.* Systemic oxygen deficiencies: the respirator brain. In: Minckler, J. (Ed.) Pathology of the Nervous System. McGraw-Hill Book Company, New York. 2:1583–1617, 1972.

290. *Linder, Hanack, Heberer, Loew, Wiemers.* Todeszeichen und Todeszeitbestimmung. Chirurg. 29:196–197, 1968.

291. *Lindgren, S., Petersen, I., Zwetnow, N.* Prediction of death in serious brain damage. Acta. Chir. Scand. 134:405–416, 1968.

292. *Liudkovskaia, I.G., Popova, L.M.* Morphology and pathogenesis of "brain death" in stroke, Arkh. Pthol. 40:48–54, 1978.

293. *Lister, J.* By the London post. The phenomenon of waiting lists—Clinical and legal death—Hazards of jogging, N. Engl. J. Med. 298:955–956, 1978.

294. *Lobstein, A., Tempe, J.D., Payeur, G.* La fluoroscopie rétinienne dans le diagnostic de la mort cérébrale. Docum. Ophthal. 26:349–358, 1969.

295. *Loeb, C.* L'apporto dell electroencefalografia al problema della cosiddetta morte cerebrale. Rass. Clin. Sci. 1st Biochem. Ital. 45:193–197, 1969.

296. *Lorenz, R.* Kriterien der Hirntätigkeit in lebensbedrohenden Zuständen—ein Beitrag zur Frage des zentralen Todes. Acta. Neurochir. 20:309–329, 1969.

297. *Lundervold, A.* Electroencephalographic changes in a case of acute cerebral anoxia unconscious for about three years. Electroenceph. Clin. Neurophysiol. 6:311–315, 1954.

298. *MacMillan, V., Siesjö, B.K.* Critical oxygen tension in the brain. Acta Physiol Scand. 82:412–414, 1971.

299. *Manaka, S., Sano, K.* Study of stationary potential (SP). II. Its value in various animals and its use for the estimation of cerebral death. Brain Nerve 24:1573–1582, 1972.

300. *Mankert, J.F.* Should the law define brain death? Hosp. Prog. 60:6, 10–11, 1979.

301. *Manning, W.H., Vogel, H.J.* The case for "brain death" legislation. A response to the critics, Minn. Med. 62:121–127, 1979.

302. *Mantz, J.M., Kurtz, D., Otteni, J.C., Rohmer, F.* EEG aspects of six cases of severe barbiturate coma. Electroenceph. Clin. Neurophysiol. 18:426, 1965.

303. *Mantz, J.M., Lobstein, A., Jaeger, A.* L'oeil dans le diagnostic de la mort cérébrale. Ann. Anesth. Franc. 15:95–100, 1974.

304. *Mantz, J.M., Tempe, J.D., Jaeger, A., Kurtz, D., Lobstein, A., Mack, G.* Silence éléctrique de vingt-quatre heures au cours d'une intoxication massive par 10 g de pentobarbital. Hemodialyse. Guerison. Presse. Med. 79:1243–1246, 1971.

305. *Marasasa, Y.* Fundamental and clinical studies on pulsatile echoencephalography under acute intracranial hypertension. J. Wakayama Med. Soc. 24:59–83, 1973.

306. *Marshall, T.K.* Premature burial. Medicoleg. J. 35:14–21, 1967.

307. *Masland, R.L.* When is a person dead? Resident and Staff Physician 21:49–52, 1975.

308. Massachusetts General Hospital. Optimum care for hopelessly ill patients. New Eng. J. Med. 295:362–364, 1976.

309. *Masshoff, W.* Zum Problem des Todes. München, Med. Wschr. 110:2473–2482, 1968.

310. *Matakas, F., Cervos-Navarro, J., Schneider, H.* Experimental brain death. J. Neurol., Neurosurg. and Psych. 36:497–508.

311. *Maynard, C.D., Witcofski, R.L., Janeway, R., Cowan, R.J.* "Radioisotope Arteriography" as an adjunct to the brain scan. Radiology 92:908–912, 1969.

312. *McCaman, B., Hirsh, H.L.* Brain death: legal issues. Heart Lung 8:1098–1102, 1979.

313. *McCormick, W.F., Halmi, N.S.* The hypophysis in patients with coma dépassé ('respirator brain'). Amer. J. Clin. Path. 54:374–383, 1970.

314. Medical Royal Colleges and their Faculties (Conference), Diagnosis of death. Lancet 1:261–262, 1979.

315. *Meek'ren, J.* Observationes medico-chirurgical. Amsterdam, H. & T. Bloom 6pl. 392 pp., 1682.

316. *Messerschmitt, J., Gamain, J., Faille, N.* Etude hematologique des comas dépassés. Ann. Anesth. Franc. 15:61–67, 1974.

317. *Milhaud, A., Ossart, M., Gayet, H., Reboulot, M.* L'épreuve de débrancher en oxygene test de mort cérébrale. Ann. Anesth. 15:73–79, 1974.

318. *Milhaud, A., Riboulot, M., Gayet, H.* Disconnecting tests and oxygen uptake in the diagnosis of total brain death. Ann. NY Acad. Sci. 315:241–251, 1978.

319. *Miller, J.R., Myers, R.E.* Neurological effects of systemic circulatory arrest in the monkey. Neurology 20:715–724, 1970.

320. *Mills, D.H.* Statutory brain death. JAMA 229:1225–1226, 1974.

321. *Mills, D.H.* More on brain death. JAMA 234:838, 1975.

322. *Minami, T., Ogawa, M., Sugimoto, T., Katsurada, K.* Hyperoxia of internal jugular venous blood in brain death. J. Neurosurg. 39/4:442–447, 1973.

323. *Mishkin, F.* Determination of cerebral death by radio-nuclide angiography. Radiology 115:135–137, 1975.

324. *Mitchell, O.C., De La Torre, E., Alexander, E., Davis, C.H.* The nonfilling phenomenon during angiography in acute intracranial hypertension. Report of 5 cases and experimental study. J. Neurosurg. 19:766–774, 1962.

325. *Miyazaki, Y.* On the criteria of brain death: particularly, loss of brainstem function as a most important criteria. Unpublished, presented at IX Symposium Neuroradiologicum, Göteborg: August 24, 1969.

326. *Miyazaki, Y., Takamatsu, H., Tanaka, Y., Mikami, N., Akagawa, S., Sohma, T.* Criteria of Cerebral Death. Acta. Radiol. 13:318–328, 1972.

327. *Mohandas, A., Chou, S.N.* Brain death. A clinical pathological study. J. Neurosurg. 35:211–218, 1971.

328. *Molinari, G.F.* Review of clinical criteria of brain death. Ann. NY Acad. Sci. 315:62–69, 1978.

329. *Molinari, G.F.* (in press).

330. *Mollaret, P.* Über die äussersten Möglichkeiten der Wiederbelebung: Die Grenzen zwischen Leben und Tod. München, Med. Wschr. 104:1539–1545, 1962.

331. *Mollaret, P., Bertrand, I., Mollaret, H.* Coma dépassé et necroses nerveuses centrales massives. Rev. Neurol. 101:116–139, 1959.

332. *Mollaret, P., Goulon, M.* Le coma dépassé. Rev. Neurol. 101:5–15, 1959.

333. *Montgomery, T.M.* Cited by Tebb, W. Vollum, E.P. Premature burial. London, Swan, Sonnenschen & Co. Ltd. 346 pp., 1905.

334. *Montoya, M.E., Hill, G.* EEG Recording in intensive care units. Am. J. EEG Technol. 8:85–95, 1968.

335. *Moores, B., Clarke, G., Lewis, B.R.* Public attitude towards kidney transplantation. Brit. Med. J. 1:629–631, 1976.

336. *Morison, R.S.* Death: process or event? Science 173:694–698, 1971.

337. *Moseley, J.I., Molinari, G.F., Walker, A.E.* Respirator brain: report of a survey and review of current concepts. Arch. Pathol. Lab. Med. 100:61–64, 1979.

338. *Mueller, N.* Die sekundären morphologischen Veränderungen des Gehirns nach Verletzung durch stumpfe Gewalt. Deutsche Med. Wschr. 91:1126–1131, 1966.

339. *Müller, H.R.* Zur Problematik der flechen Hirnstromkurve und der Diagnose "Hirntod" nach akuter zerebrale Anoxie. Med. Klin. 61:1955–1959, 1966.

340. *Mutuskina, E.A.* Significance of some EEG parameters in the early prognosis of the severity of injuries of the CNS following total ischemia of the brain. Pat. Fiziol. Eksp. Ter. 16:47–51, 1972.

341. *Myers, R.E., Yamaguchi, M.* Effects of serum glucose concentration on brain response to circulatory arrest. J. Neuropath. Exp. Neurol. 35:301, 1976.

342. *Nathanson, M., Bergman, P.S., Anderson, P.J.* Significance of oculocephalic and caloric responses in the unconscious patient. Neurology 7:829–832, 1957.

343. *Nedey, R., Brian, S., Jedynak, P., Arfel, G.* Neuropathologie du coma dépassé. Ann. Anesth. Franc. 15:3–11, 1974.

344. *Negovsky, V.A.* Some physiopathologic regularities in the process of dying and resuscitation. Circulation 23:452–457, 1961.

345. Netherlands Red Cross Society. Summary of the report of the Ad Hoc Committee on Organ Transplantation. 19 pp., 1971.

346. News item. Kansas City Star. November 3, 1967, p. l.

347. News item. The Boston Herald American. May 14, 1977, p. l.

348. News item. Time Magazine. June 7, 1976.

349. News item. Albuquerque Tribune. May 23, 1980, p. C6.

350. *Nicholson, A.N., Freeland, S.A., Brierley, J.B.* A behavioural and neuropathological study of the sequelae of profound hypoxia. Brain Research. 22:327–345, 1970.

351. *Nimmannitya, J., Walker, A.E.* Significance of the electroencephalogram in comatose respirator cases. Curr. Med. Digest 36:189–200, 1969.

352. *Nordlander, S., Wiklund, P.E., Asard, E.* Cerebral angioscintigraphy in brain death and in coma due to drug intoxication. J. Nucl. Med. 14:856–857, 1973.

353. *Oden, T.C.* The Quinlan decision; five commentaries. Beyond an ethic of immediate sympathy. Hastings Cent. Rep. 6:12–14, 1976.

354. *Oftedal, S.I., Bachen, N.E., Lundervold, A., Sawhney, B.B.* The use of evoked potentials in evaluation of brain death. Electroenceph. Clin. Neurophysiol. 30:273, 1971.

355. *Oldendorf, W.H., Kitano, M.* Radioisotope measurement of brain blood turnover times as a clinical index of brain circulation. J. Nucl. Med. 8:570–587, 1967.

356. *Olsson, Y., Hossmann, K.-A.* The effect of intravascular saline perfusion on the sequelae of transient cerebral ischemia. Acta. Neuropath. 17:68–79, 1971.

357. *Opitz, E., Schneider, M.* Über die Sauerstoffversorgung des Gehirns und den Mechanismus von Mangelwirkungen. Ergebn. Physiol. 46:126–260, 1950.

358. *Ossart, M., Gayet, H., Milhaud, A.* Technique de maintien en survie des coma dépassés. Ann. Anesth. Franc. 15:123–131, 1974.

359. *Ouaknine, G.* Bedside procedures in the diagnosis of brain death. Resuscitation 4:159–177, 1975.

360. *Ouaknine, G.E.* Cardiac and metabolic alterations in brain death: discussion paper. Ann. NY Acad. Sci. 315:252–264, 1978.

361. *Ouaknine, G., Kosary, I.Z., Braham, J., Czerniak, P., Nathan, H.* Laboratory criteria of brain death. J. Neurosurg. 39:429–433, 1973.

362. *Ouaknine, G., Kosary, I.Z., Ziv, M.* Valeur du test calorique et de l'électronystagmographie dans le diagnostic du coma dépassé. Neuro-Chirurgie 19:407–414, 1973.

363. *Paillas, J.E.* Les critères de la mort du donneur dans les transplantations d'organes. Marseille Med. 107:369–380, 1970.

364. *Pampiglione, G., Chaloner, J., Harden, A., O'Brien, J.* Transitory ischemia/anoxia in young children and the prediction of quality of survival. Ann. NY Acad. Sci. 315:281–292, 1978.

365. *Pampiglione, G., Harden, A.* Resuscitation after cardiocirculatory arrest: prognostic evaluation of early electroencephalographic findings. Lancet 1:1261–1265, 1968.

366. *Parvey, L.S., Gerald, B.* Angiographic diagnosis of brain death in children. Pediatr. Radiol. 4:79–82, 1976.

367. *Paulson, G.W., Wise, G., Conkle, R.* Cerebrospinal fluid lactic acid in death and in brain death. Neurology 22:505–509, May, 1972.

368. *Pearcy, W.C., Virtue, R.W.* The electroencephalogram in hypothermia with circulatory arrest. Anesthesiology 20:341–347, 1959.

369. *Pearson, J., Korein, J., Braunstein, P.* Morphology of defectively perfused brains in patients with persistent extracranial circulation. Ann. NY Acad. Sci. 315:265–271, 1978.

370. *Pendl, G., Ganglberger, A., Stenbereithner, K., Tschakaloff, C.* Cerebraler Zirkulationsstillstand in Korrelation mit EEG und pO2AVD-Untersuchungen. Acta. Radiol. 13:329–333, 1972.

371. *Penin, H., Kaeufer, C.* The dissociated brain death: clinical and electroencephalographic criteria for determination of death. Minn. Med. 51:1563–1567, 1968.

372. *Penin, H., Kaeufer, C.* Der Hirntod, Todes zeitbestimmung bei irreversiblem Funktionsverlust des Gehirns. Georg Thieme Verlag. Stuttgart, 1969.

373. *Pevsner, P.H., Bushan, C., Ottesen, O.E., Walker, A.E.* Cerebral blood flow and oxygen consumption: an on-line technique. Hopkins Med. J. 128:134–140, 1971.

374. *Pines, N.* The ophthalmoscopic evidence of death. Brit. J. Ophthalm. 15:512–513, 1931.

375. *Pitts, L.H., Kaktis, J., Caronna, J., Jennett, S., Hoff, J.T.* Brain death, apneic diffusion oxygenation, and organ transplantation. J. Trauma 18:180–183, 1978.

376. *Plum, F.* Brain histology in anoxic encephalopathy after short period of apnea. JAMA 214:1895, 1970.

377. *Plum, F.* The clinical problem: How much anoxia-ischemia damages the brain? Arch. Neurol. 29:359–360, 1973.

378. *Plum, F., Posner, J.B.* Diagnosis of stu-

por and coma. Philadelphia, F.A. Davis Co., 2nd Edit. ix + 286 pp., 1972.

379. *Pope Pius XII.* The prolongation of life. An address of Pope Pius XII to an international congress of anesthesiologists. The Pope Speaks 4:393–398, 1958. (Acta Apostolicae Sedia. 49:17, 1957.)

380. *Posner, J.B.* Coma and other states of consciousness: the differential diagnosis of brain death. Ann. NY Acad. Sci. 315:215–227, 1978.

381. *Powner, D.J.* Drug-associated isoelectric EEGs—a hazard in brain-death certification. JAMA 236:1123, 1976.

382. *Powner, D.J., Fromm, G.H.* The electroencephalogram in the determination of brain death (letter). N. Engl. J. Med. 300:502, 1979.

383. *Powner, D.J., Grenvik, A.* Triage in patient care: from expected recovery to brain death. Heart Lung 8:1103–1108, 1979.

384. *Pribram, H.F.W.* Angiographic appearances in acute intracranial hypertension. Neurology 11:10–21, 1961.

385. *Prior, P.F., Maynard, D.E., Sheaff, P.C., Simpson, B.R., Strunin, L., Weaver, E.J.M., Scott, D.F.* Monitoring cerebral function: clinical experience with new device for continuous recording of electrical activity of brain. Brit. Med. J. 2:736–738, 1971.

386. *Prochazka, M.* Knekterym diagnostickym problemum takzvane mozkove smirti. Cas. Lek. Ces. 112:1166–1168, 1973.

387. *Prochazka, M., Ciganek, L.* The diagnostic value of midriasis in cerebral death. Phronesis, Rev. Neurol. Neurocir. Psiquiat. 10:321–324, 1973.

388. *Prochazka, M., Dornetzhuberone, M., Papiernikova, E.* Angiographic evidence of brain circulatory arrest in cerebral death. Bratisl. Lek. Listy. 61:595–599, 1974.

389. *Rabkin, M.T., Gillerman, G., Rice, N.R.* Orders not to resuscitate. New Eng. J. Med. 295:364–366, 1976.

390. *Råadberg, C., Såoderlundh, S.* Computer tomography in cerebral death. Acta Radiol. (Suppl.) 346:119–129, 1975.

391. *Rangel, R.A.* Computerized axial tomography in brain death. Stroke 9:597–598, 1978.

392. *Rappaport, Z.H., Brinker, R.A., Rovit, R.L.* Evaluation of brain death by contrast-enhanced computerized cranial tomography. Neurosurgery 2:230–232, 1978.

393. *Ray, C.D., Vogel, P.* Instrumentation for deep brain implantation for the diagnosis of death. Conf. Neurol. 34:112–126, 1972.

394. *Riehl, J.L., McIntyre, H.B.* Reliability of the EEG in the determination of cerebral death: report of a case with recovery of an isoelectric tracing. Bull. Los Angeles Neurol. Soc. 33:86–89, 1968.

395. *Riishede, J., Ethelberg, S.* Angiographic changes in sudden and severe herniation of brain stem through tentorial incisure. Report of five cases. Arch. Neurol. Psychiat. 70:399–409, 1953.

396. *Riishede, J., Jacobsen, H.H.* Cerebral angiography in the diagnosis of brain death. (in preparation).

397. *Roelofs, R.* Some preliminary remarks on brain death. Ann. NY Acad. Sci. 315:39–44, 1978.

398. *Rosoff, S.D., Schwab, R.S.* The EEG in establishing brain death. A 10-year report with criteria and legal safeguards in the 50 states. Electroenceph. Clin. Neurophysiol. 24:283–284, 1968.

399. Royal Colleges and Faculties in the United Kingdom. Br. Med. J. 2:1187–1188, 1976. Lancet 2:1069–1070, 1976.

400. *Rubin, R., Brennan, R.E., Jacobs, G.B., Hubbard, J.H., Wille, R.L.* Cerebral death. J. Med. Soc. N.J. 75:825–828, 1978.

401. *Sadler, A.M., Sadler, B.L.* The Uniform Anatomical Gift Act: a two-year report. New Eng. J. Med. 283:156, 1970.

402. *Safar, P.* Gauging: evaluation of salvability. In: *Resuscitation: Controversial Aspects.* Safar. P. Ed.) Springer-Verlag, Berlin: 50–52, 1963.

403. *Salah, S., Valenćak, E., Kulsha-Lissberg, E., Grunert, V.* Dans quelle measure l'angiographie est-elle un paramètre de la mort cérébrale. Neurochirugie 18:49–52, 1972.

404. *Sament, S., Alderete, J.F., Schwab, R.S.* The persistence of the electroretinogram in patients with flat isoelectric EEGs. Electroenceph. Clin. Neurophysiol. 26:121, 1969.

405. *Schafer, J.A., Caronna, J.J.* Duration of apnea needed to confirm brain death. Neurology (Minneap.) 28:661–666, 1978.

406. *Scharfetter, F.* Die Zeichen des unabwendbaren Todes und die Frage, wann die Wiederbelebung als aussichtslos einzustellen ist. Z Allgemeinmed. 45:830–834, 1969.

407. *Scharfetter, C;, Schmoigl, S.* Zum isolektrischen Enzephalogram (Aussagewert nach Aussetzen der Spontanatmung). Deutsche Med. Wschr. 92:472–475, 1967.

408. *Schewe, G., Adebahr, G.* Sekundaer-

scháden am Gehirn bei Schädeltrauma. Z Rechtsmed. 67:129–146, 1970.

409. *Schneider, H.* Zur Feststellung des Hirntodes Dtsch. Med. Wschr. 94:2404–2405, 1969.

410. *Schneider, H.* Der Hirntod. Begriffsgeschichte und Pathogenese. Nervenarzt. 41:381–387, 1970.

411. *Schneider, H., Masshoff, W., Neuhaus, G.A.* Klinische und morphologische Aspeckte des Hirntodes. Klin. Wschr. 47:844–859, 1969.

412. *Schneider, H., Matakas, F.* Pathological changes of the spinal cord after brain death. Acta Neuropath. 18:234–247, 1971.

413. *Schneider, H., Matakas, F., Simon, R.S.*, Hypertension intracrânienne et infarctus ischemique total du cerveau. Neuro-Chirurgie 18:159–70, 1972.

414. *Schneider, M.* The metabolism of the brain in ischemia and hypothermia. In: *Metabolism of the Nervous System.* Edited by Richter, D., Pergamon Press, New York, 238–244, 1957.

415. *Schneider, M.* Survival and revival of the brain in anoxia and ischemia. In: *Cerebral Anoxia and the Electroencephalogram.* Meyer, J.S. and Gastaut, H (Eds.). Charles C Thomas, Springfield, Illinois: 134–143, 1961.

416. *Schroeder, J.S., Rider, A.K., Stinson, E.B., Shumway, N.E.* Cardiac transplantation: review of seven years' experience. Transplantation Proc. 8:5–8. 1976.

417. *Schulz, H.* Practical determination of the irreversible loss of all cerebral functions (Brain death), Desk Neurol. Neurochir. 41:166–172, 1978.

418. *Schuster, H.P., Busch, H., Busch, G., Niemczyk, H., Baum, P., Knolle, J., von Ungern-Sternerg, A., Lang, K.* Zur Problematik des dissoziierten Hirntodes bei Patienten eines internistischen Intensivpflegezentrums. Deutsche Med. Wschr. 94:2118–2121, 1969.

419. *Schwab, R.S., Potts, F., Bonazzi, A.* EEG as an aid in determining death in the presence of cardiac activity (ethical, legal and medical aspects). Electroenceph. Clin. Neurophysiol. 15:147–148, 1963.

420. *Schwartz, B.A.* Non-existent or imperceptible EEG activity. Electroenceph. Clin. Neurophysiol. 29:531, 1970.

421. *Schwartz, B.A., Vendrely, E.* Un des problèmes poses par le diagnostic du coma dépassé: EEG nul et diametre pupillaire. Rev. Neurol. 21:319–323, 1969.

422. *Scott, D.F., Prior, P.F.* Reversible death. Lancet 1:188–189, 1971.

423. Segal, cited by Carroll (89).

424. *Shakespeare, W.* Hamlet, Act I, Sc. 2, line 129.

425. *Shalit, M.N., Beller, A.J., Feinsod, M., Drapkin, A.J., Cotev, S.* The blood flow and oxygen consumption of the dying brain. Neurology 20:740–748, 1970.

426. *Shapiro, H.A.* Brain death and organ transplantation. J. Forensic Med. 15:89–90, 1968.

427. *Siesjo, Nilsson, L., Rokeach, M., Zwetnow, N.N.* Energy metabolism of the brain at reduced cerebral perfusion pressures and in arterial hypoxaemia. In: *Brain hypoxia*, edited by J. B. Brierley and B. S. Meldrum. London: William Heinemann Medical Books, Ltd., Philadelphia, J. B. Lippincott Co., 8:79–93, 1971.

428. *Silverman, D.* Criteria of brain death. Science 170:1000, 1970.

429. *Silverman, D.* Cerebral death: the history of the syndrome and its identification. Ann. Intern. Med. 74:1003–1005, 1971.

430. *Silverman, D., Masland, R.L., Saunders, M.G., Schwab, R.S.* Irreversible coma associated with electrocerebral silence. Neurology 20:525–533, 1970.

431. *Silverman, D., Saunders, M.G., Schwab, R.S., Masland, R.L.* Cerebral death and the electroencephalogram. Report of the Ad Hoc Committee of the American Electroencephalographic Society on EEG Criteria for Determination of Cerebral Death. JAMA 209:1505–1510, 1969.

432. *Simpson, K.* The moment of death: a new medico-legal problem. Acta. Anaesth. Scand. Suppl. 29:361–379, 1968.

433. *Sims, J.K.* Pupillary diameter in irreversible coma. New Eng. J. Med. 285:57, 1971.

434. *Sims, J.K., Bickford, R.G.* Non-mydriatic pupils occurring in human brain death. Bull. Los Ang. Neurol. Soc. 38:24–32, 1973.

435. *Sims, J.K., Billinger, T.W.* Types of EKG artifact seen during EEG—electrocerebral silence. The Westwind 11:89–94, 1971.

436. *Sims, J.K., Casler, J.A., Billinger, T.W., Aung, M.H., Shattuck, C.M., Fleming, N.I., Bickford, R.G.* The human electroretinogram in alert volunteer and in brain death patients; new recording techniques. Proc. San Diego Biomed. Symp., 1972.

437. *Sims, J.K., Hagan, S.L.* The persistence of the M-Echos in the A-mode

echoencephalograms of patients demonstrating 'irreversible coma with brain inactivity.' Bull. Los Ang. Neurol. Soc. 38:138–146, 1971.

438. *Smith, A.J.K., Penry, J.K. (Eds).* Brain Death, NINDS Bibliography Series No. 1, Government Printing Office, Washington, D.C., DHEW Publication No. (NIH) 73–347, 19, pp.1–30, 1972.

439. *Smith, A.J.K., Walker, A.E.* Cerebral blood flow and brain metabolism as indicators of cerebral death. The Johns Hopkins Med. J. 133:107-119, 1973.

440. Societé d'EEG et de Neurophysiologie Clinique de Langue Française. Recommendations provisoires de la Commission de la Societé d'E.E.G. et de Neurophysiologie clinique de langue française chargée de'étudier les signes E.E.G. de la 'mort cérébrale'. Rev. Neurol 121:237-238, 1969.

441. *Sokoloff, L.* The action of drugs on the cerebral circulation. Pharm. Rev. 1-85, 1959.

442. *Soloveichik, A.* Jewish law and time of death (letter). JAMA 240:109, 1978.

443. *Solnizky, O.* Death of the brain: a vital diagnostic factor in organ transplantation. Georgetown Med. Bull. 23:94-103, 1970.

444. *Spann, W.* Vorstellungen zur Gesetzgebung über den tatsächlichen Todeszeitpunkt. Münch. Med. Wschr. 111:2253-2255, 1969.

445. *Spann, W., Kugler, J., Liehardt, E.* Tod und elektrische Stille im EEG. Münch. Med. Wschr. 109:2161-2167, 1967.

446. *Spann, W., Liebhardt, E.* Reanimation und Festsellung des Todeszeitpunktes. Münch. Med. Wschr. 108:1410-1414, 1966.

447. *Spudis, E.V.* Brain death (letter). JAMA 239:1958-1959, 1978.

448. *Starr, A.* Brain-stem responses in brain death. Brain 99:543-545, 1976.

449. *Steegmann, A.T.* The neuropathology of cardiac arrest. In: Minckler, J. (Editor), Pathology of the Nervous System. Mc-Graw-Hill Book Co., New York. 1:1005-1029, 1968.

450. *Steinwall, O.* Extracranial monitoring of intravenously given ^{75}Se selenomethionine in the diagnosis of brain death. Acta Neurol. Scand. (Suppl.) 51:497, 1972.

451. *Stochdorph, O.* Pathologie des Ruckenmarks. In: Handbuch der Neurochirugie. Springer, Berlin, Heidelberg and New York. 7:238-304, 1969.

452. *Stodlmeister, R., Wilmanns, I., Koenig, A., Gabriel, W.* EEG-Registrierung beim Hirntod. Prakt. Anaesth. 13:446-449, 1978.

453. *Suter, C., Brush, J.* Clinical problems of brain death and coma in intensive care units. Ann. NY Acad. Sci. 315:398-416, 1978.

454. *Sweet, W.H.* Brain death (editorial), N. Engl. J. Med. 299:410, 412, 1978.

455. *Tabaddor, K., Gardner, T.J., Walker, A.E.* Cerebral circulation and metabolism at deep hypothermia. Neurology 22:1065-1070, 1972

456. *Tendler, M.D.* Cessation of brain function: ethical implications in terminal care and organ transplant. Ann. NY Acad. Sci. 315:394-397, 1978.

457. *Tentler, R.L., Sadove, M., Becka, D.R., Taylor, R.C.* Electroencephalographic evidence of cortical 'death' followed by full recovery: protective action of hypothermia. JAMA 164:1667-1670, 1957.

458. *Teraura, T., Handa, H., Mori, K.* Determination of death: electrophysiological background. Int. Anesth. Clin. 13:235-244, 1975.

459. *Thienes, C.H., Haley, T.J.* Clinical Toxicology. Ed. 5. Philadelphia, Lea & Febiger, 459 pp., 1972.

460. *Toennis, W., Frowein, R.A.* Wie lange ist Wiederbelebung bei schweren Hirnverletzungen möglich? Mschr. Unfallheilk. 66:169-190, 1963.

461. *Toole, J.F.* The neurologist and the concept of brain death. Perspect. Biol. Med. 14:599-607, 1971.

462. *Towbin, A.* The respirator brain death syndrome. Human Pathology 4:583-594, 1973.

463. *Trillet, M.* Comas prolonges et 'mort du cerveau' post-traumatiques. Aspects cliques et anatomiques. Acta. Psychiat. Belg. 70:378-418, 1970.

464. *Trojaborg, W., Jorgensen, E.O.* Evoked cortical potentials in patients with "isoelectric" EEGs. Electroenceph. Clin. Neurophysiol. 35:301-309, 1973.

465. *Troupp, H.* Ventricular fluid pressure recording after severe brain injuries. Eur. Neurol. 11:227-34, 1974.

466. *Troupp, H., Heiskanen, O.O.* Cerebral angiography in cases of extremely high intracranial pressure. Acta. Neurol. Scand. 39:213-223, 1963.

467. *Tsementzis, S.A.* Significance of the ventricular fluid pressure wave form in the diagnosis of cerebral circulatory arrest and brain death. Acta Neurochir. 40:191-202, 1978.

468. *Tyson, R.N.* Simulation of cerebral

death by succinylcholine sensitivity. Arch. Neurol. 30:409-411, 1974.

469. *Ueki, K., Takeuchi, K., Katsurada, K.* Clinical study of brain death. Presentation No. 286, Fifth International Congress of Neurological Surgery, Tokyo, Japan, 1973.

470. *Uematsu, S., Walker, A.E.* Pulsatile cerebral midline echo and brain death. Johns Hopkins Med. J., 134:383-390, 1974.

471. *Uematsu, S., Smith, T.D., Walker, A.E.* Pulsatile cerebral echo in diagnosis of brain death, J. Neurosurg. 48:866-875, 1978.

472. U.S. Navy Department. Determination of cerebral death or electroencephalographic silence. Bumed. Instruction 5360.24, April 15, 1974.

473. Vanderbilt Law Review—Legal problems in donations of human tissues to medical science. Vanderbilt Law Review 21:352-374, 1968.

474. *Vanderhaeghen, J-J, E.R., Logan, W.J.* The effect of the pH on the in vitro development of Spielmeyer's ischemic neuronal changes. J. Neuropath. Exp. Neurol. 30:99-104, 1971.

475. *van Till-d'Aulnis de Bourouill, H.A.H.* Legal aspects of the definition and diagnosis of death. Handb. Clin. Neurol. 24:787-828, 1976.

476. *Veatch, R.M.* Defining death: the role of brain function, JAMA 242:2001-2002, 1979.

477. *Veath, R.* Brain death. Hastings Center Report. 11:10-13, 1972.

478. *Veghelyi, P.V.* Ethics of intensive treatment. Anaesthesist. 19:468-472, 1970.

479. *Veith, F.J.* Brain death and organ transplantation, Ann. NY Acad. Sci. 315:417-441, 1978.

480. *Velasco, M., Lopez-Portillo, M., Olvera-Radiela, J.E., Velasco, F.* EEG y registros profundos en casos de coma post traumatico irreversible. Arch. Inv. Med (mex.) 2:1-15, 1971.

481. *Vigouroux, R.P.* Colloque sur les états frontières entre le vie et la mort. Marseille Chir. 18, 194, 1966.

482. *Vigouroux, R.P., Naquet, R., Chamant, U.H., Baurand, C., Chou, M., Vigoureux, M.* Nouvel essai de classification des états frontières entre la vie et la mort. Neuro-Chirurgie 18:53-56, 1972.

483. *Vigouroux, R.P.* Between life and death. Handbook EEG Clin. Neurophysiol. 12(8):95-99, 1975.

484. *Visser, S.L.* Two cases of isoelectric EEG. Electroenceph. Clin. Neurophysiol. 27:215, 1969.

485. *Vlahovitch, B. In Gros, C.* Les critères circulatoires et biologiques de la mort du cerveau. Neuro-Chirurgie. 18:9-48. (p. 26), 1972.

486. *Vlahovitch. B., Boudet, C.* La circulation ophthalmique dans les comas dépassès. Images obtenues par l'angiographie carotidienne sous pression. Arch. Opthal. 33:123-128, 1973.

487. *Vlahovitch, B., Frèrebeau, P., Kuhner, A., Billet, M., Gros, C.* Les angiographies sous pression dans la mort du cerveau avec arrêt circulatoire encéphalique. Neuro-Chirurgie 17:81-96, 1971.

488. *Vlahovitch, B., Frèrebeau, P., Kuhner, A., Stopak, B., Allais, B., Gros, C.* Arrêt circulatoire intracranien dans la mort du cerveau: Angiographie avec injection sous pression. Acta. Radiol. 13:334-349, 1972.

489. *Voisin, C., Wattel, F., Scherpereel, P.H.* Apport de l'étude biochemique liquide cephalorachidien au diagnostic de mort cérébrale. Ann. Anesth. Franc. 15:87-93, 1974.

490. *Wald, A., Hass, W., Ransohoff, J., Wood, D.H.* Wald tutorial: Experience With A Mass Spectrometer System for Blood Gas Analysis in Humans, J. Assoc. Adv. Med. Instru. 5:325-342, 1971.

491. *Wald, A., Hass, W.K., Siew, F.P., Wood, D.H.* Continuous Measurement of Blood Gases *In Vivo* by Mass Spectrography. Med. Biol. Eng. 8:111-128, 1970.

492. *Walker, A.E.* The death of a brain. Johns Hopkins Med. J. 124:190-201, 1969.

493. *Walker, A.E. Cerebral Death.* In: The Nervous System. (Vol. II) Edited by Tower, D.B. New York, Raven Press, pp. 75-87, 1975.

494. *Walker, A.E.* Invited editorial. The neurosurgeon's responsibility for organ procurement. J. Neurosurg. 44:1-2, 1976.

495. *Walker, A.E.* Advances in the determination of cerebral death, Adv. Neurol. 22: 167-177, 1979.

496. *Walker, A.E.* Ancillary studies in the diagnosis of brain death, Ann. NY Acad. Sci. 315:228-240, 1978.

497. *Walker, A.E.* Pathology of brain death, Ann. NY Acad. Sci. 315:272-280, 1978.

498. *Walker, A.E., Diamond, E.L., Moseley, J.* The neuropathological findings in irreversible coma. J. Neuropathol. Exp. Neurol. 34:295-323, 1975.

499. *Walker, A.E., Molinari, G.F.* Sedative drug surveys in coma. How reliable are they? Postgrad. Med. 61:105-109, 1977.

500. *Walsh, G.O.* Small apparatus to mon-

itor for possible or impending electrocerebral silence. Bull. Los Angeles Neurol. Soc. 39:154–157, 1974.

501. *Waltregny, A., Bonnai, J., LeJeune, G.* Morte cérébrale et homotransplant. Critères utilisés pour établir rapidement le diagnostic de coma dépassé. Rev. Neurol 122:406–411, 1970.

502. *Wasmuth, C.F.* The concept of death. Ohio State Law. J. 30:32–60, 1969.

503. *Wawersik, J.* Kriterien des Todes unter dem Aspekt der Reanimation. Chirurg. 39:345–348, 1968.

504. *Webster, H.D., Ames, A.* Reversible and irreversible changes in the fine structure of nervous tissue during oxygen and glucose deprivation, J. Cell Biol. 26:885–909, 1965.

505. *Webster, N.* New International Dictionary, 2nd Edition, Springfield, Mass., G & C Merriam Co. 3214 pp., 1951.

506. *Wecht, C.H.* Protocol for the determination of death. Penn. Med. 72:17-20, 1969.

507. *Wecht, C.H.* Brain death diagnosed by ultrasonic technique. Int. Med. and Diagnosis News. 3:1, 1970

508. *Weiner, I.H.* Death criteria. JAMA 222:86, 2 Oct. 1972.

509. *Welby, H.* Mysteries of life, death, and futurity. Cited by Arnold (25).

510. *Wertheimer, P., Jouvet, M., Descotes, J.* A propos du diagnostic de la mort du système nerveux—dans les comas avec arrêt réspiratoire traités par respiration artificielle. Presse Méd. 67:87–88, 1959.

511. *Wexler, J.* Pupil size and irreversible coma. New Eng. J. Med. 285:526, 1971.

512. *Wilder, A.* Burying alive—a frequent peril. Cited by Marshall (306).

513. *Wilkus, R.J., Chatrain, G.E., Lettich, E.* The electroretinogram during terminal anoxia in humans. Electroenceph. Clin. Neurophysiol. 31:537–546, 1971.

514. *Windle, W.F., Jacobson, H.N., Robert de Ramirez de Arellano, M.L., Combs, C.M.* Structural and functional sequelae of asphyxia neonatorum in monkeys (Macaca mulatta). Res. Pub. Ass. Res. Nerv. Ment. Dis. 39:169–182, 1962.

515. *Winter, A.* The Moment of Death. Charles C. Thomas, Springfield:84, 1969.

516. *Winter, A.* Life and death decisions, Springfield, Illinois, C.C Thomas 1980, xiii + 71 pp

517. Working Party. The removal of cadaveric organs for transplantation. A Code of practice. Health Depts. Great Britain and Northern Ireland, H.M. Stationery Office 1979, 36pp

518. *Yamada, R., Katsurada, K., Sugimoto, T.* Hemodynamic defect in patients with severe head injury. Injury, 6:351–357, 1975.

519. *Yamada, R., Minami, T., Tahara, I., Ogawa, M., Katsurada, K., Sugimoto, T.* "Brain death"—hemodynamic aspects. Brain Nerve. 25:257–264, 1973.

520. *Yamauchi, Y., Sugitani, Y., Katsurada, K.* An application of echoencephalography to non-perfused and luxury perfused human brain, Med. J. Osaka Univ. 24:101-109, 1973.

521. *Yashon, D., Wagner, F.C., Locke, G.E., White, R.H.* Clinical, chemical and physiological indicators of cerebral nonviability in circulatory arrest. Trans. Amer. Neurol. Ass. 95:31–35, 1970.

522. *Yashon, D., Wagner, F.C., White, R.J., Albin, M.S., Locke, G.E.* Intracranial pressure during circulatory arrest. Brain Res. 31:139–150, 1971.

523. *Yoneda, S.* Relationship between the duration of cerebral circulatory arrest and the recovery of electrocorticogram and cerebral blood gas analysis: An indicator for clinical criteria of brain death. Arch. Jap. Chir. 42:157–168, 1973.

524. *Zander, E., Cornu, O.* Les critères de la morte cérébrale. Revue critique de 90 cas. Schweiz. Med. Wschr. 100:408–414, 1970.

525. *Zander, E., Rabinowicz, D.T., Tribolet, N.* Etude anatomo-clinique de la mort cérébrale. Schweiz. Med. Wschr. 101:1225–1234, 1971.

526. *Zattoni, J., Fritz, D., Giasotto, G.* Correlazione fra indici liquorali del metabolismo cerebrale e spettro di pôtenza dell EEG nel coma profondo verso la morte cerebrale. Boll. Socital. Biol. Sper. 47:798–801, 1971.

527. *Zwetnow, N.N.* Multifokala intracerebrala injektioner av ädelgasisotop-en ny klinisk metod för fastställande av hjärndöd. Nordisk Med. 85:675–676, 1971.

Subject Index

Author Index

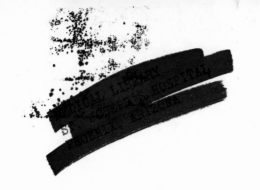